Basic Steps
in
Planning Nursing
Research

Pamela J. Brink, R.N., Ph.D, F.A.A.N.

Marilynn J. Wood, R.N., Dr. P.H.

UCLA School of Nursing
Los Angeles, California

Basic Steps in Planning Nursing Research:

From Question to Proposal

Duxbury Press
North Scituate, Massachusetts

Library of Congress Cataloging in Publication Data

Brink, Pamela J.
  Basic steps in planning nursing research.

  Bibliography: p.
  Includes index.
  1. Nursing—Research. I. Wood, Marilynn, J.,
joint author. II. Title.
TR81.5.B74   610.73'072   77-20160
ISBN 0-87872-174-6

Duxbury Press
A Division of Wadsworth Publishing Company, Inc.

L.C. Cat. Card No.: 77-20160
ISBN 0-87872-174-6
Printed in the United States of America
    4 5 6 7 8 9 — 82 81 80

Contents

Preface

Any research project begins with the planning phase. This involves finding one problem and only one problem for study; asking a question about that problem; intensively reviewing the literature on the problem; deciding how to solve the problem; planning how to collect the data; deciding which analysis best suits the data; deciding how to best protect the rights of the sample; and then writing a proposal that is clear to anyone not familiar with all of the thinking that went into the plan.

Once the proposal is written and approved by a committee on the protection of human rights, data collection can begin. Data collection is primarily a "doing" phase; it is the actual legwork of research, done either by the researcher or a research assistant. If the proposal is clear and precise, anyone can collect the necessary data.

After data are collected, the researcher must try to make some sense of it—analyze, think about, and organize the data into some reasonable and explainable package. The data analysis plan in the proposal is used as the basis for this phase, but may be altered to allow for unanticipated results. The phrase "The best laid plans of mice and men . . ." can be applied to the analysis phase. Unless the research design were a very rigidly controlled experimental design, there will be data that do not fall within the analysis plan. This is the time for rethinking the entire research process.

The final step in research design—writing up the results—is the end product of all the foregoing. This phase requires writing skills. Although the research itself may have evolved in fits and starts, the written report must be an even statement of procedures, discoveries, and conclusions. The report should be logical, consistent, readable, intelligible, and carefully documented throughout. Clarity and completeness are critical to this report, since other researchers may want to replicate the research.

Although based upon the previous stages, each phase requires different skills, levels of information, and solutions to the problems that inevitably arise. No one research text can possibly do justice to each phase. When a text attempts to cover each and every part of the research process, something is usually left out to allow for a full discussion of another. If, for example, the text attempts a full exposition on all possible types of data analysis methods, little space may be left in the text for the proposal. On the other hand, if each phase is handled adequately, the size of the volume would look something like an unabridged dictionary, requiring a desk of its own to hold it up. Finally, depending upon the problems researched, the number of research methods used by the physical, social, and health sciences is enormous. Since nursing draws from many fields for its research base, an adequate coverage of all possible methods and their analyses would provide material for another tome.

With these issues in mind, and with the objective of writing a text for the beginning researcher, that is, someone who has never had a research course or experienced research before, the only logical solution would be to have a series of books on the different levels and stages of the research process, since no single book would do justice to the field.

This book is written as an introduction to the research process and deals solely with the beginning phase of research—the research plan. The book begins with finding a research topic and ends with the written research proposal. This book cannot, and does not, claim to stand alone as an exhaustive treatment of all phases of the research process. It is a beginner's book and treats the planning process as an art in and of itself. All attempts at sophistication have been ruthlessly blue-pencilled, replaced by simple words and terms easily understood. The simplicity of approach, however, should not be confused with simple-mindedness.

This book is intended specifically for the student who is taking an introductory course in research, whether on an undergraduate or graduate level. Most introductory research courses are based on the planning phase of research, but few introductory research texts devote adequate space to this portion of the research process. This text is designed to fill that gap. Recommended readings are listed at the end of each chapter that provide more in-depth treatment on that particular subject.

The basic thesis of this book is that research is only as good as its plan, and that a well-conceived plan is of immeasurable assistance throughout the rest of the process. But planning takes thought, library research, organization, and a lot of hard work. Showing the student where to find information, what kinds of organization are possible, what to look for in the literature, and how to ask a researchable question in the first place, should provide a clearer picture of what a research project entails and how to go about it.

LEVELS OF RESEARCH	STEM QUESTION	CONCEPTUAL FRAMEWORK/ KNOWLEDGE BASE	PURPOSE	DESIGN	METHOD	ANALYSIS	ANSWER
LEVEL I	What Where When Who	Little or no knowledge of topic May not have a conceptual base	Declarative statement	Situational control Exploratory/ descriptive Case study	Unstructured observation Open-ended interviews and questionnaires Participant observation Unwritten available data Written available data	Content analysis Descriptive statistics Graphs Charts Tables	Description Concepts Categories of variables Categorized processes
LEVEL II	What are the Differences/ relationships Between/among	Prior knowledge of topic, but action of variables cannot be predicted Has a conceptual base	Question	Both situational and investigator control Descriptive survey	Structured observation Open and closed (mixed) questionnaires and interviews Available written data Projective tests	In addition— Inferential statistics Correlational analysis Differences between means	Hypothesis Explanation of relationship of between/among variables in conceptual framework
LEVEL III	Why If-then	Full knowledge of topic; action of variables can be predicted Has a conceptual or theoretical base	Hypothesis	Investigator control Survey/ explanatory Explanatory-/ experimental	All available structured methods	All available statistical tests and/or analyses	Support or reject hypothesis, thereby adding to the knowledge base of the conceptual or theoretical framework

I.

What Is Research?

Ever since the first person said, "there must be a better way," human beings have been asking questions about the universe and trying to improve the quality of life. The invention of the wheel, the electric light, and the automobile all resulted from painstaking thought, trial and error, problem solving, and research to find that better way. The same is true of new surgical techniques and new drugs —both are products of a need to improve the human environment.

The human mind is always questioning. As children we asked, "Why is the grass green? What makes the sun go down? Why does my dog have fur? Why do I always fall down instead of up?" Most adults would answer the questions with "because," which satisfied us as a statement of fact. But if we found a different opinion in every answer, or if we heard "I don't know," we kept asking questions because as human beings we had to know.

The purpose of research is to answer questions, whether they arise from a practical need or simple curiosity. But not all questions can or need to be answered by research. Some questions already have answers. Others, by their very nature, can only elicit an opinion, for example, "How many angels can dance on the head of a pin?" Other questions can be satisfied with an immediate answer: "What's the fastest way of getting to your house?" Questions asking "What should I do?" or "Where should I go?" require opinions and therefore are not suitable for research.

What, then, is a research question?

A research question is an explicit query about a problem or issue that can be challenged, examined, analyzed, and will yield useful new information. The researcher restates the query in the form of a position and then tests that position to arrive at conclusions that can be generalized and can themselves be questioned and retested. Answers to research questions add to our general knowledge. They can be used by other people in other places because the answers are valid no matter who asked the question or where the answer was found. This is the critical feature of research findings—they must be facts, not opinions.

Identical duplication of research questions, while possible, is rare. Similar questions occur over and over again and give rise to replication studies which can be useful in themselves, but identical questions that are significant and usable are extremely unusual. If you have thought of a specific, clear research question, you can be assured that in all probability no one else has asked exactly that same question. Whether your question explores an entirely new avenue of thought, or examines an area that has been explored before, the exact question is yours.

If you can support your position and document your procedure, you have done something unique in that no one else has thought of your exact question.

The research question is a reflection of the opinions and ideas of the researcher. Thus, the types of questions and the problems chosen for study are as varied as the people who choose them. Some people are interested in minute detail, others, in the overall picture. Some are interested in people, others in mechanical objects. Some are interested in ideas, others in actions. All such topics are amenable to research. But they must all be subjected to the research question.

In order to do research, the first step is to find a topic to research. Where can topics be found and how do you know they are researchable?

RESEARCH TOPICS

Finding a research topic isn't as hard as it seems at first. Once you develop the ability of looking for researchable topics, they appear everywhere. Experienced researchers become so good at spotting research problems that they usually have at least a dozen ideas waiting to be investigated. But finding topics can be intimidating at first.

Where do you look for research topics?

The most fruitful area for research topics is your own thoughts, observations, and experiences. What have you been reading lately? Who have you been talking to and what did you talk about? Where have you been? When you read a book, you may find yourself disagreeing with the author, or you may feel that the author didn't prove the point to your satisfaction. You may think of several counterarguments to refute the author's position. You may find yourself annoyed with the author's bias. Whenever you disagree with something you have read, you have the beginnings of a research topic. If you have experienced a similar reaction to a conversation or someone's behavior, you also have a potential research topic.

That research topics should arise out of these areas is natural. You know something about the subject. You have some facts or opinions that contrast with another's point of view. You read something that contradicted the position you just heard. You were taught a slightly different approach. Your personal experiences did not agree with the generalizations being made. Or you may have found a flaw in the logical development of the argument. Wherever the source of your disagreement, you may have found yourself frustrated by the fact that you could not positively prove that the other person was wrong. This is the basis for the research question.

The second aspect of topic selection is that you wouldn't be irritated or frustrated unless you were interested in the subject being discussed. Just how interested you are depends upon how long your reactions linger. If you immediately forget your irritation, you aren't that interested. If it keeps nagging at you, you probably have an interest that will sustain you throughout the research. Since you will need a subject that will interest you long enough to complete the research process, use this rule of thumb to gauge your interest level.

Knowing enough about your topic and being interested in it are basic requirements for selection.

How do you know if your knowledge is extensive enough? Take stock of what you do know. Where did you learn it? If your entire stock of information is based on accidental, personal experience, you may find that this amount of knowledge is not enough to sustain you. If, on the other hand, you have talked to a number of people about this subject, have been reading in the area, and if your personal observations have reinforced what you have read and heard, you certainly know enough to begin.

If you want to do research on nursing supervisors and their leadership strategies but your entire stock of information is based upon being a staff nurse, you don't know enough to do a study of supervisors. What you do know about is being a staff nurse, who is subjected to different administrative strategies. If you have talked to other nurses about different supervisors, and have read about supervision and how it is best accomplished, you are well on your way to do research on the nurses' perceptions of various administrative strategies. But you would have some difficulty with the administrators' perceptions and decisions on supervisory strategies because that's not really where your interest lies. You might, in fact, bias your research against the supervisor simply because your interest is in the nurses. Knowing enough about your subject means that you know what you are specifically interested in, that is, you must identify your point of view.

Judging the extent of your knowledge about a particular subject depends upon how specific the problem is. The more general the problem, the more people share facts and opinions about the problem. Suppose your research problem was nursing and your research question was "What is nursing?" You wouldn't be proving anything one way or another, since a general description of nursing already exists. On the other hand, a question such as "What is primary care nursing and how effective is it in health maintenance?" requires more specific information about primary care nursing. You would have to read about the subject, find out the arguments for and against this specialty, and use the information to formulate your opinion, which must be susceptible to testing with new facts.

Fortunately, you have been studying nursing and command a wealth of information that you may not realize you have. This knowledge can provide sources for research problems. In the area of patient care, you know about a variety of pathologies and medical interventions. You also know that there are different nursing care strategies based on which health agency the patient comes to and for what health problem. Have you formed any opinion on how to improve patient care in any of these areas? Do you think you would be able to document it? If so, how? You may have noticed that certain patients within the same agency and with the same problems receive different care. You wonder if this is because of the patient or the staff. You have been reading about stereotyping and wondered if patients were being stereotyped and treated according to the label.

Theoretical issues provide an entire area of research topics. Role theory offers innumerable ideas whether relating to singular roles, such as the sick role, or studies of roles in interaction, such as the patient role versus the nurse role. Concepts concerning the patient's psychological reactions, such as grief, loss, denial, alienation, and immobility, can be applied to almost any patient situation for testing.

Testing assessment and intervention strategies is another field for exploration. How these strategies are used and developed, and who uses them and for what, are areas open to divergent opinion and fact-building. Behavior modification, crises intervention, and implosive therapy are interventions that need to be tested on a variety of patients in a variety of settings.

No single theory, hunch, opinion, or even fact is ever totally researched. There is always room for further challenges and explorations. The less that is known about a particular subject, the more work needs to be done. The more work that has been done, the more refinement is necessary.

If you have an idea but you don't know to what extent the subject has been covered, if at all, the simplest way to find out is to go to the card catalogue in the library. The fewer books on the subject, the less that has been done. Since texts normally cover the research to date, the more books, the more that has been done. Look up related ideas and concepts in the same way. Then go to the cumulative indexes and hunt for your idea there. Magazine and journal articles present the most recent developments in the field. Finally, ask for a computer search of your topic. As your search narrows, so will your topic.

Now that you have a general idea about research topics and where to find them, the next step is to ask a question about the topic.

WHAT MAKES A RESEARCH QUESTION?

Any question that yields hard facts that will help to solve a problem, produce new research, add to theory, or improve nursing practice is a researchable question. A research question that yields opinion rather than facts can lead to an interesting article or essay but is not researchable. Research deals with facts, with observable phenomena in the real world. A question that will provide answers that explain, describe, identify, substantiate, predict, or qualify is a researchable question.

For this reason, research must be *usable*. Because research deals with the real world, the findings should add to knowledge that can be used by other researchers, theorists, or practitioners. Whether the question deals with improving patient care, administration, services, or educational strategies, the answer should actually help to improve those areas. Whoever reads the published report with the intention of using the findings, relies on the researcher having been *ethical* in writing the report—that the facts as presented are true and based on a reliable study. If findings are to be used, the study must be honest and reliable.

To be of use, research questions should be *now* questions. No matter how good the research is, if the society does not need or want the research findings, they will be ignored. Therefore, questions should be relevant to the issues of the day. In nursing, clinical questions, in particular, are *now* questions. Nursing desperately needs the answers to clinical questions that are practical and immediately usable.

Research questions need to be *clear*. Fuzzy questions yield fuzzy answers. A fuzzy answer is neither usable nor ethical. Therefore, the clearer the question, the clearer the answer and the more usable in clinical settings.

Finally, a researchable question lends direction to the rest of the research report. If the research question were about an event, directive questions would ask: What happened? When did it happen? In what way did it happen? To whom did it happen? What difference did it make, now that it happened? These questions demand more of an answer than a simple *yes, no,* or *maybe.* Without some movement in the question, it is just a "sitter," without impetus or direction. *Sitters* are questions that elicit answers such as, "Yes, that's interesting," or "And then what?," or even worse for the researcher, "Well, now, what are you going to do about it?"

Now is the time to examine the research question in more detail, to show what it does, how it is written, what the parts are, and what each part of the question does. Since many people find research a difficult process and feel overwhelmed before they are through, they stop before they have any sense of completion or accomplishment. One of the reasons for this is that they either did not have a clearly stated question to work with, or they chose a highly complex question as their first effort. Both of these are guaranteed to produce a very hopeless feeling before the plan is even completed. As a research novice, starting with a simple, clearly stated question practically assures you of seeing the research plan through to the finished proposal. A simple question is less likely to lead to a complicated research design than a complex question, which assuredly will. As you progress through this book you will find that this statement is very true, but for the moment, just accept the fact that the simpler the question, the greater the chance of satisfaction from this, your first effort.

Everything in your research plan depends on your question. It is the point you want to make, to explore, to describe, or to know, stripped clean of any superfluous verbiage. It is your research purpose stated in one simple, comprehensive sentence. To arrive at this point, you will have to ferret out all interesting but irrelevant distractions, seek out the very essence of what you want to know, and move from a very broad subject to the one specific point you want to make. Now let's build research questions and see how the process works.

Writing Research Questions

Although there are no hard and fast rules for writing research questions, there are still some guidelines that you can follow, depending on the subject you have chosen.

There are two basic components to every question—the subject (or topic) being examined, and the question itself. Simple questions have one topic and one question. *Who stole the cookies?* The question is *who* and the topic is *stolen cookies.* The question could as easily have been *When do bedsores occur?* The question is *when* and the topic is *occurrence of bedsores.* In research, every simple question must be answered, no matter how complex the question, since complex questions must be reduced to their component simple questions. For example:

When do bedsores occur and what causes them?

Three distinct simple questions can be derived from this one complex question:

1. When do bedsores occur?
2. What causes bedsores?
3. What is the relationship between the cause and onset of bedsores?

In the first question, the question was *when,* while the last two questions were *what* questions. In addition, there are now three topics: 1) occurrence of bedsores; 2) cause of bedsores; and 3) relationship between onset and cause of bedsores.

Since research requires an answer to each simple question within a complex statement, the first rule-of-thumb is to *reduce your idea to a simple question.*

The type of question you ask about your topic is the basis for the design of your research plan. As such, your question is action-oriented, demanding some activity on your part to answer. Whether you must go to the library, go out into the community to question people, observe a group of children playing, or work in a laboratory to find the answer, your particular activity is inherent in the question you have asked. For this reason, the second rule-of-thumb is *ask an active question.*

You may have noticed that in published reports of research, the author presented a statement or a hypothesis rather than a question. This is perfectly appropriate to a finished report or a published study, as you will see later, but at the beginning of the research plan you need something that will provide direction. Since you are concerned with the planning phase of the research project, you are dealing in future tense, what you will and won't do when you start to collect your data. A question rather than a statement is called for in this instance. Notice the difference in the following sentences:

Mastectomy has an effect on women.
What are the reactions of women to mastectomy?

In the first sentence, the statement is a declaration of fact requiring no action on anyone's part. The question, on the other hand, demands an answer. The following series of statements and questions illustrates the differences between a question and a statement.

1. Age has an effect on convalescence.
   What effect does age have on convalescence?
2. Black women have smaller babies than white women.
   What is the difference in size of babies born to white women versus black women?
3. Ice water increases heart rate.
   What effect does ice water have on heart rate?

As you can see, a statement of fact demands no action whereas a question does.

You will find as you start to write questions that some do not require action. Any question that can be answered by a *yes* or *no* is not an action-oriented question. These questions are *stoppers.* They stop action because the question has been answered, obviating the need to do any research. Questions that begin with *should* or *could* are also stoppers; they elicit opinions, not facts.

Should nurses wear white uniforms?
Should everyone have a yearly x ray?
Should patients bathe in the morning?

Everyone has an opinion on each of the above questions. If you can assume that your population would answer *yes, no,* or *I don't know* to these questions, and have a ninety-five percent chance that you would be right, then you don't need to do research to find the answer. Try rewriting each of the *should* questions into action questions that require investigation to find the answer and notice the difference in the way the question is phrased.

Inactive verbs are also stoppers; they can usually be answered by yes or no as well as should or could. Although inactive verbs provide more direction than should or could questions, they, too, lead to opinions rather than action.

> Do nurses neglect patients?
>
> Do patients respond to pain in the same way?
>
> Do patients with coronary heart disease tend to keep their clinic appointments more regularly than other types of patients?

Look at each of these questions in relation to their basic components, the topic and the question. In the first example the topic is *nurses neglect patients,* and the question is *do. Do* doesn't imply much action, does it? Change *do* to *what,* and the question becomes *What nurses neglect patients?* If *what* were exchanged for *do* in the second question, the same thing would happen. *What patients respond to pain in the same way?* The answers can no longer be simple *yes* or *no* opinions; they require some form of action to find the answer.

As you are trying to write your questions as simply as possible, don't be discouraged if you find yourself writing *yes* or *no* questions— even the most advanced researchers find themselves slipping into stoppers. Your first task is to try to write your question as simply as possible, which may entail writing a complex question and breaking it down into its simple component questions first. Once you have done that, you can look at the type of question you have asked and separate the question from your topic. The third rule-of-thumb is to *substitute measurement questions for opinion questions.*

A *measurement question* requires some form of action or measurement for an answer. Measurement questions imply that the researcher will have to observe something, participate in something, or question someone in order to arrive at an answer. The way the question is worded specifies how the researcher intends to measure the quantity or quality of the topic. Measurement, in the research sense, means examining an abstract idea to derive a concrete answer. Whether the answer is in numerical form or a description, it is observable and concrete. A measurement question, then, provides some direction for the researcher to answer the question in a measurable (concrete) form.

The basic measurement questions that will readily substitute for opinion questions are: *who, what, when, where,* and *why.*

Go back to the *should* questions and see which of these measurement questions will replace them; which could be inserted in front of the *should;* and which would have to be rephrased or rewritten to use one of the measurement questions. Do the same thing with the *do* questions. Notice how, in each case, the answer will differ because the question has changed.

> Should nurses wear white uniforms?
> Why should nurses wear white uniforms?
> Why do nurses wear white uniforms?
> What nurses wear white uniforms?
> Where do nurses wear white uniforms?
> When do nurses wear white uniforms?

All of the answers to the questions about nurses and white uniforms have been changed. The *why should* question is a study of opinions about wearing white uniforms. *Why do* asks for causes for wearing white uniforms. *What* wants to know the relationship between types of nurses and uniform color. *Where* asks if there are differences in situations that call for color coding of uniforms. *When* is a question about time. And because the questions are different, the answers will differ, too.

Beginning with a measurement question as the basic question, you are asking that your topic stimulate and direct the rest of your research proposal. Not only does the measurement question insure some action on your part, it also tells you in which direction you must go to answer the question.

Now that you have your basic question and your topic written down as a simple question (or a series of simple questions), the next step is to rewrite your topic. This step is not as alarming as it might seem. If you have written a simple topic such as *nurses neglect patients*, the revisions can be done very rapidly. The only change that needs to be made with this topic is to rearrange the word order in the sentence to *patients are neglected by nurses.* In the first question the emphasis is on the nurses, while the second focuses on the patients. Now put the topic back together with the stem questions and note the difference in the types of answers the questions require.

Stem Questions	*Topic*
What	nurses neglect patients?
What	patients are neglected by nurses?
Why do	nurses neglect patients?

Why are	patients neglected by nurses?
When do	nurses neglect patients?
When are	patients neglected by nurses?

In each case the emphasis placed in the topic alters the emphasis in the answer. *Rewriting the topic by reordering the words* is the fourth rule-of-thumb. By reordering the emphasis, you explore the possible ramifications of your topic before you decide which question to ask.

Examining the Components of the Question

Now that you have a general idea about research topics and some guidelines for asking questions about the topic, your next step is to look at each component of your question in more detail. There are two basic components to your question, the *stem question* and the *topic*. Both components must be examined separately to see what they do and how they will affect the rest of your plan.

The Stem Question.   Since all research requires some plan for collecting information in order to answer the question, the way you ask the question is the way you will answer it. A Chinese philosopher once said, "The answer is in the question." This statement is just as true in research as it is in philosophy. But in research, the method of obtaining the answer is expressed in the stem question.

In the section on writing research questions, you were introduced to the differences between measurement stem questions (who, what, where, why, when) and opinion stem questions (inactive verbs and yes/no questions). You probably noticed that when each stem question was attached to a topic, the entire direction of the question changed. You also no doubt concluded that any stem question could be attached to a topic. The decision as to which stem question to attach to a topic is based entirely on your judgment, but you should understand the uses of stem questions and the answers they elicit.

Before deciding which stem question to use, you need to know that stem questions fall into three distinct groups. Group I stem questions (what, where, when, who) are simple stems that require a description for an answer. Group II stems are *what* questions such as those in Group I but requiring a more complex answer. Group II stems require descriptive answers about the *relationship* between two or more things—not descriptions of the things themselves. *Why* and *if-then* questions fall in group III. Answers to Group III questions will either explain *why* or attempt to prove cause-and-effect.

What questions always require a descriptive answer. Whenever you ask *what* about anything, the answer will always be in the form of a description. *What happened?* The answer will describe the events that took place. *What caused?* The answer will describe the cause. *What is the relationship between?* The answer will describe the relationship between the things named. No matter to what topic you apply the *what* question, you will always have to describe what you find. Whether you ask about past, present, future events, people, things, or beliefs, the type of answer remains the same.

Notice the difference between the following questions:

What nurses use the nursing process in their daily practice?
What is the difference between nurses who use the nursing process and nurses who don't use the nursing process in their daily practice?

As you can readily see, there is a distinct difference in these two types of *what* questions. The first one is a simple question of a simple topic. The second one restates the first in a more complex form that asks for a comparison between nurses. This progression depends on the amount of knowledge available to you as the investigator. To ask the second question, you must already know the answer to the first; for example, what nurses use the nursing process.

What questions require two levels of information—simple description and comparative description. For this reason, the chart in the front of this book has separated *what* questions into two different levels.

Other types of comparative *what* questions would look like this:

"What is the similarity between . . ."
"What are the significant differences among . . ."

And so on. Just keep in mind when you are writing a *what* question that there are two kinds. Start with a simple *what* question before you try to ask a comparative *what* question.

When questions always involve time answers, whether in seconds, minutes, hours, days, years or phases. *When* questions demand that you know what time period you are interested in. Whether you are examining causes, outcomes, events, or how people structure time, you will need to be specific about what time period you are dealing with.

Like *what* questions, *when* questions will have descriptive answers but of a specific nature. Events, people, stages, processes, and ideas can be described in a time context. *When did? When will? When do? When are?* —these questions are answered with a description.

Where questions obviously require a description of location, whether geographic or abstract. *Where is an item located? Where does a thing begin? Where will a change occur? Where* questions necessitate specific descriptions of place.

Answers to *who* questions will always involve descriptions, counting, categorizations, and/or biographies. Questions asking who did, said, believed, wrote will require detailed demographic information. When you write a *who* question you will need to keep in mind categories such as age, sex, ethnicity, educational level, occupation, health, roles, and so on.

How questions should always be used with discretion. Try other stem questions before you resort to a *how* question. The reason for this reservation is that *how* questions fit into both Group I and Group II levels.

The *how* questions that fall into Group I include: *How many? How much? How often?* These are simple questions that demand simple numerical answers.

But *how* questions are also process questions requiring a description of a means to an end. *How* questions in this group ask: *In What way? In what manner? For what reason? By what means? To what extent? From what cause? Under what conditions? How* questions of this type must be worded for maximum clarity. The word *how* is so versatile that the answers cannot be categorized as easily as those for the Group I—the complexity of answers is much greater than for simple questions, yet causes are not named. Rather the answers describe a process.

Why questions compel an explanatory answer. *Why* questions elicit causes to explain a fact, theory, or observation. They are highly sophisticated questions based on a thorough understanding of how the subject of the study operates. Whenever you know the effect but not the cause, you will ask a *why* question. *Why is the grass green? Why is the sky blue? Why does lack of iodine in the diet cause goiter?* To answer a *why* question, you need a well-developed research method and statistical analysis in order to prove your point. The highest level of research question is the *why* question.

If-then questions, like *why* questions, require sophisticated answers and the use of statistics to prove that the answer did not happen by chance. Like *why* question, *if-then* questions fall in Group III stem questions because of the type of answer they require. *If-then* questions are manipulative questions: If this changes, then what will happen? If I as the researcher change something in the situation, then will something else in the situation change as a result? As the researcher, you manipulate the IF clause, and observe and describe the resulting THEN occurrences.

Examples of *if-then* questions are as follows: If this is changed in this way, then how often will change occur in that? If cold solutions are used in tube feedings, then what changes will occur in peristalsis as a result?

If-then questions, like *why* questions, are based on greater knowledge than the questions in either Group I or Group II. If you don't know anything about your research topic, begin by asking a Group I question. As your knowledge about the topic increases, the research will require a higher level of question.

Refer to the chart in the front of this book and observe the division of stem questions according to levels. If you look at the other columns in the chart, you can see that the level of stem question directs the rest of the research plan, including the purpose, the design, and the answer. The chart is a handy guide to the relationship between the question and the answer. It also provides a check list for you to use to make sure your research plan stays on the same level of questioning.

The levels of stem questions refer to the level of knowledge about the topic; the level of knowledge refers to the amount and type of research that has been done on the topic. If there has been a great deal of research done on a topic, a *what, when,* or *where* stem question is inappropriate. On the other hand, if little research has been done on the topic, a *why* or *if-then* stem question is far too advanced to begin with.

As we go on in this book, we will show you how the level of question affects the complexity of the research plan.

The Topic.   Whether you have decided to do research on a theory, a concept, another researcher's findings, or something you have observed or thought about, you will quickly discover that some topics are easier to specify than others. Research deals with facts, with *observable* phenomena. The further away your topic is from observable phenomena, the harder it is to define it for research. But the point remains that you must specify your topic if you are to research it.

How is this accomplished?

After you have written your simple question(s) with one stem question and one topic, separate your stem question from the topic.

Stem Question	*Topic*
What are	nurses' attitudes towards patients?

Your topic is now *nurses' attitudes towards patients.* Look at each word in the topic separately. You should be able to define how you intend to use each word in your research. These definitions should conform to the requirement of research—that the factors can be observed and measured on some scale. This is called a *working definition.*

Starting with *nurses,* use your list of measurement questions and ask these questions of *nurses. What* nurses do you intend to study? *Where* are those nurses? *When* do you intend to study them? *Who* are they (demographically)? *Why* did you choose these nurses over others for your study?

Since you will be studying nurses' attitudes toward patients, nurses are your population. You cannot possibly study the entire population of nurses in the United States, so you must sample the population. The way you sample will be based on the answers to the preceding questions. You are fortunate in that your sample is named in the question; not all questions include the sample but have to be found outside of the question. (Further discussion on the sample comes under the section on research design.) With the exception of the *why* questions, your answers to all of the measurement questions will provide you with a working definition of *nurses* that might look like this:

> *Nurses:* Registered nurses from all levels of basic preparation and all ethnic groups, between the ages of 25 and 35, employed in an acute-care hospital of not less than 250 beds for at least 6 months on the evening shift.

You now have a working definition of which nurses you intend to study. It is clear from your definition who you are including and who you are excluding. Your decisions may have been arbitrary, but you had some idea of where you would find your nurses, what nurses you wanted to include, and why you selected those nurses over others. These nurses are now observable; they no longer belong to that broad, amorphous group called *nurses*.

The next word in the topic is *attitudes*. Like nurses, attitudes must be defined. What attitudes are you going to study? Positive, negative, apathetic? Whose attitudes will you study? This has already been answered—nurses'. When and where do nurses have these attitudes? How are these attitudes expressed? Why do nurses have these attitudes?

Since attitude is the real focus of your study, you must attempt a *working definition* of the word. Ask the same measurement questions you asked of nurses. Since attitudes are not directly observable in and of themselves, you must decide whether you are interested in what the nurses say their attitudes are, or in how their attitudes are expressed through observable behavior. You find you will have to go to the library and read about attitudes so that you can eventually write a very specific definition. For the moment, though, you may write your working definition something like this:

> *Attitudes:* Verbal statements of negative feelings.

The third word in your statement is *patients*. Again, just as with nurses and attitudes, apply the measurement questions to the amorphous word *patients*. Here you need to have some notion about what kinds of patients would possibly elicit negative feelings in nurses. Just as with nurses, you have to narrow your patient population to an observable group. What patients will you study? Where will the patients be found? (They should be available either in the same place as the nurses or where nurses will have come in contact with them to have developed an attitude about them.) Why you have selected these patients and not others is a very critical question to answer. For the purpose of discussion, let's write a working definition of *patients:*

> *Patients:* Alcoholic patients admitted for simple detoxification as inpatients in acute-care hospitals.

You now have the three words in your topic narrowed down to working definitions that meet the requirements of being observable and measurable in some way. The question itself has become clearer and more specific.

Stem question	*Topic*
What are	Registered nurses' negative attitudes toward alcoholic patients?

As a result, you now have a *new* topic and will have to write working definitions for all the new words found in this topic. You have already defined nurses as registered nurses; therefore, no further definition is required. You have defined attitudes as negative feelings; therefore, you must define what you mean by *negative* in observable terms. In the same way, you will have to define *alcoholic* according to some observable measures such as diagnosis on the chart or admission for alcoholic detoxification.

The point here is that in specifying your topic, *every* word requires a working definition at the outset, and each word used to further refine or clarify your original terms must also be given a working definition. Notice that you did not have to add every word in your definition to your new question. Only those words that *narrowed down* the topic needed to be added. But every word, without exception, had to be defined.

The whole point to this exercise is not to cause you more work, but rather to enable you to clarify just exactly what you mean by your question. The best way to clarify your own thoughts is to define each word in your topic by simply stating how you are going to use the word in your study. Secondly, try to state specifically how you intend to observe or measure your terms, what you will include or exclude, and so on. These are *your* working definitions—beginning statements of what you intend to study. These definitions are not final; they are simply guides for your literature review. But the more specific you are at this stage, the more you will thank yourself later on.

Rewriting the Question.   Once you have narrowed your topic as far as you can at this point, put your written topic back together with your stem question to form your final working question. Is this the question you really want to ask about your topic? Do you need to change your stem question as a result of your revised topic? Put your topic on one side of a piece of paper, and list all the possible stem questions you can think of on the other side. By a process of elimination, select the stem question that best fits what you really want to know about your topic.

Stem Questions	*Topic*
What . . . have . . .	registered nurses' . . .
What kinds of . . . have . . .	negative attitudes toward
How many . . . have . . .	detoxifying alcoholic pa-
How often do . . . have . . .	tients
How intense are . . .	
When do . . . have . . .	
Why do . . . have . . .	
On what wards do (where) . . . have	

You now have a working, researchable question that will carry you through the rest of your research plan. Keep your question and your working definitions together in a workbook for easy reference since you will be referring to them constantly and making alterations and additions. Your question is the blueprint for the rest of your study.

Be Interested In Your Idea

A solid research topic is always worth doing and doing well, but research is only as good as the time and effort put into it. Don't choose a research topic because it looks easy to do. All research requires painstaking thought and a good deal of writing and reading before the proposal is finished. You might get by with a minimal amount of effort, but you will have lost an opportunity to really explore something that is meaningful to you. On the other hand, don't choose a topic that is so grandiose that it can't possibly be done simply to impress your instructor or supervisor. You may attract attention, but that isn't a solid basis for learning research.

Choose a topic that really interests you, something that will keep you going back, and back again, to the literature, your notes, or your own thoughts. This does not mean that you must retain the first thought you had when you began to write your question. On the contrary you may find one small aspect of the larger problem that you had never thought of before. But this will not occur without your being intimately involved in the larger topic to begin with. This kind of involvement is necessary if your research project is to be successful.

RECOMMENDED READING

Abdellah, Faye G. and Levine, Eugene. *Better Patient Care Through Nursing Research*. New York: MacMillan Co., 1965.

Downs, Florence S., and Newman, Margaret A. *A Source Book of Nursing Research*. Philadelphia: F. A. Davis Company, 1973.

Ellis, Rosemary. "Asking the Research Question." *Issues in Research: Social, Professional, and Methodological*. Selected Papers from the American Nurse's Association Council of Nurse Researchers Program Meeting, August 22–24, 1973, pp. 31–35.

Verhonick, Phyllis J. *Nursing Research I*. Boston: Little, Brown and Company, 1975.

II.

From Question to Problem

Throughout the entire first chapter, the words *research topic, research problem,* and *research subject* were used interchangeably. This was done quite deliberately. In research, the research problem stands by itself as the moving force behind the research plan. It is developed from the research question and is the final and complete synthesis of everything you have thought, read, argued over, and written. It substantiates what you propose to do and why. Prior to this point, however, you have been talking about problems that occur in real life, situations that need solutions, topics or ideas that interest you, and subject areas that you want to explore. As they were used in the first chapter, the terms *subjects, topics* and *problems* were a less sophisticated order of thinking than the research problem for your proposal.

In research, the research problem is the full exposition of your idea that you want to research. The problem statement or the problem definition—however you prefer to think of it—is a logical progression of ideas and arguments about your research idea. The problem introduces your topic, explains its importance, condenses facts and theories about the topic, and then in a final decisive section justifies conclusively your choice of topic. The full problem answers all of the possible *who, what, where, when,* and *why* questions that anyone not involved in your project would ever dream of asking. And those answers are firm, so definitive, that there are no loose ends, no gaps, and no fuzziness in the reader's mind.

In essence, the *research problem* is an *essay* about your research topic. An essay is a statement of opinion, substantiated by facts, that proves the position taken on a subject. A good essay offers an orderly progression of ideas that carries the reader through to the logical conclusion. Research problems should be written in the same way as good essays.

As many research reports begin with the research problem, you may be wondering why this book began by asking a question. The question serves the same purpose in research as the thesis serves for an essay. In an essay, the thesis is "the author's opinion boiled down to one arguable statement."* The research question does the same thing—it is the entire research design boiled down to one measurable question. Just as the entire essay is built on the thesis statement, the entire research proposal is built from the research question. Building a research plan from your research question is the sole object of this book.

In the previous chapter, you were introduced to some of the functions of the research question and pinning down your subject. In this section, you will be refining your question into its clearest, most

---

*See Lucille Payne Vaughn, *The Lively Art of Writing* (New York: Mentor Books, 1965), p. 25.

concise form and moving into the development of the research problem.

CLOSING IN ON YOUR PROBLEM

Although there are any number of ideas that you could have chosen to do research on, most research questions can be grouped into a few primary categories: theory, concepts, observed situations, prior research, and tool development. Each category has different requirements for solution and different end products. Each has its practical aspects, drawbacks, literature, and logic. Each has its supporters and its detractors. But all are valid. No one is "better" than another; it's simply a matter of what interests you the most. Some people always start with questioning a theory, some always start by questioning an observed situation. It's really a matter of "goodness of fit" between the researcher and the topic. If you want to question a clinical situation that has been bothering you, don't drop the idea because it's not a theory question. On the other hand, don't just attach any old theory to your question; your question will direct you to the appropriate one. Conversely, if you are a theorist at heart, your question will direct you to the appropriate situation to study; not every situation will suit your theory. The point is, your question will tell you where you are going and what you are going to do. Remember that it's your question and no one else's; how you develop it is *your* responsibility.

Now let's take some research topics and divide them into groupings:

Observations
Some patients refuse medications.
Some patients are called demanding.
Some call lights aren't answered.
Mastectomy seems to affect some women more than others.
Detoxification programs don't always work on heroin addicts.

Behaviors
Listening
Eating
Touching
Distancing
Avoiding
Talking

Concepts
Anxiety
Powerlessness
Grief

Hopelessness
Denial

Theories
Loss theory
Role theory
Alienation theory
Theories of aggression
Psychopathological theories
Theories of change
Learning theory
Germ theory
Biorhythmical theory
Ethological theory
Systems theory

Each category of topic classifies a different order of phenomena. *Observations* arise from real-life situations that can be seen, smelled, touched, tasted or heard by any individual. Often an observation is stated as a generalization about repeating occurrence. It is the generalization that is usually tested in the research project.

Behaviors are specific types of observations that can be seen and thought about. In nursing, research is frequently based on observed behaviors of patients or nurses. However, since behavior is frequently seen as purposive or goal-directed, analysis of behavioral intent is more abstract and more removed from reality than a direct personal observation. Therefore, research on behavior is more abstract than research on observations and should be treated as a different level of abstraction.

Concepts are single ideas, often expressed in a single word, that represent two or more interrelated ideas. A concept can represent a single group of observations or facts that are closely linked to one another in a distinguishable pattern. Research can be done on one concept and its component parts, but the interconnections between the ideas, which form the basis for the study, must be discussed.

Theories are explanation of two or more interrelated concepts; as such, they are the farthest removed from reality or direct observations. Theories are abstractions of processes, interactions, and observations.

As you can see, each successive category moves farther and farther away from the requirements of being observable and measurable because the level of abstraction increases. Since research deals with observable phenomena that can be described, classified, or explained, the closer the research topic is to observable fact, the easier it will be to pin down the elements in the research question. Not only are observations easier to pin down, you are more familiar with them since you have made one or more of these observations for yourself.

At the opposite extreme, theories are the most difficult to pin down since they are the farthest removed from observable facts. You may be familiar with the general idea of the theory and some of the work that has been done on it, but you are not as familiar or knowledgeable about theory as you are with observations. If you can refine a theory into measurable, observable terms, you should be able to pin down concepts and behaviors even more easily.

Since research requires explanation as well as observation, it will always involve some level of abstraction or theory. Whether you build your problem essay from an observation to a theory or begin with a theory and reduce it to measurable terms, you must relate theory to facts.

Since theory is more difficult to pin down than observations, let's close in on our problem by starting with theory.

THE STEP-BY-STEP PROCESS

The process of putting theory into an observable, measurable research question involves a thorough inventory of your knowledge about the theory; deciding which concepts within the theory most interest you; asking yourself which behaviors best exemplify the concept you have chosen; and, finally, choosing those observations that best represent those behaviors. Since you are narrowing down from abstraction to observation, you are moving from a generalization to a specific. Pinning down theory is a process of identifying what you want to know and filtering out all unnecessary material until you have narrowed your subject to its purest, most refined point. Let's see how it works.

Finding out What You Know

Let's say that your research question is: "In what way do patients learn their role?" Now you must define the terms in your question to determine the extent of your knowledge about the theories involved.

You know that the terms *role* and *learn* stand for major theories, and you must decide in which aspect of those words you are interested. At the same time, you need to find out just how much you know about both theories in order to have a starting point for your literature search, since you don't want to waste time going over familiar ground.

So you begin with your working definition of your terms.

You define *role* as: That group of behaviors commonly found among ill persons in a hospital setting. Suddenly you are uncomfortably aware of how far away you are from an observable, measurable definition of the term. As you look at your definition, you can see you need to define just what you mean by *that group of behaviors,* since that phrase is very vague. You also see that you need to define "ill person" more specifically; and *hospital setting* isn't exactly the clearest term, either.

What you have is a series of concepts all tied together into one word that stands for an entire theory. And you must have a working (measurable) definition of each word. You have just discovered that each concept must be broken down into its component parts, each of which must be defined in relation to some observable, measurable behavior.

So you turn to the dictionary for help.

> *Role:* A part, or character, performed by an actor in a drama; hence a part taken, or assumed by anyone.*

Each of those words must be defined as well, so you are no further along than before. In fact, you may have become somewhat confused, since a patient is not an actor in the sense that the dictionary seems to imply. So what do you do?

Return to your original definition. You are interested in three major interrelated concepts in role theory: *ill people, hospital settings,* and *grouped behaviors.* You have three areas in which to search the literature, look up definitions, plan a computer search, or seek out the reference librarian. On the other hand, you wrote working definitions of each area in order to narrow down, still further, just which aspects of the theories interest you and how much you know about each. These definitions will provide you with this information.

Asking Questions About the Theory

According to your question, you are most interested in how patients learn their role. Therefore, you must ask:

> Who teaches role and how is it taught?
> Are there different types of patient roles to be learned?
> Is the patient role easy or difficult to learn?
> Are patients satisfied or dissatisfied with their roles?
> What kind of a role is the patient role?
> What other roles interact with the patient role?

Websters New Collegiate Dictionary (Springfield Mass.: G. & C. Merriam Co., Publishers, 1959.)

Is terminal illness a role situation?

Does the diagnosis of cancer change the patient role?

How does the type of hospital the patient is in affect the patient role?

All of these questions, as well as others you may think of, will need to be answered by some aspect of role theory. You are again faced with the measurement questions of *who, what, where, why,* and *when,* this time in relation to patients and roles.

As you ask your questions and read what other people have thought or observed, take notes on the answers and opinions that you encounter. You can use index cards for your notes, making sure that you accurately cite the references to avoid having to look them up again at a later stage.

Head each card with a question, and as you read, jot down notes on the answers and cite the author, title, publication date, and page number. This will provide you with a series of cards with answers to each of your questions. When you are finished, group your cards under the appropriate questions. Then examine each set of answer cards and decide which answers you agree with—or feel most comfortable with—and separate them from the other cards. You now have a beginning outline of those aspects of role theory in relation to ill patients that most interest you.

Looking up Interrelated Ideas

Since a concept is made up of at least two ideas, and a theory, of at least two concepts, there is always the possibility that at least one of the ideas inherent in the theory will lead to an entirely different concept or even a different theory. Therefore, as you search the literature, look up all relevant related concepts and ideas. You may find a fruitful new line of thought that leads you away from your original idea or reinforces your approach to your question. Look carefully at these ideas and accept or reject them on the basis of knowledge, not hunch.

This search will also tell you whether you have eliminated too many ideas in the initial development of your question. Use this aspect of the literature review to clarify your topic, making sure you have left out nothing important and are not including anything irrelevant or superfluous.

Outlining

Starting with the major heading, begin to break down your theory into the component parts that fit your question. (Remember that each

major heading has at least two minor contrasting headings under it.)
This outlining process helps you become more specific about what
aspect of the theory interests you. Also, you are identifying areas within
the theory that appear to be interrelated.

As you outline, include only those aspects of the theory that you
agree with and exclude those areas that you consider to be irrelevant or
unimportant. From this will emerge your specific point of view. However, don't throw away the other arguments; keep them handy where
you can refer to them when you are developing your full and final
problem.

Role
    I. Role types
       A. Patient roles
          1. In-patient
          2. Out-patient
          3. Convalescent
          4. Terminal
             a. patient doesn't know
             b. patient knows
                1) recently told
                2) has known for some time
          5. Short-term
          6. Long-term
          7. Emergency
       B. Staff roles
       C. Family roles
       D. Sick roles
    II. Role learning
   III. Achieved versus ascribed roles
   IV. Role distance
    V. Role behaviors
   VI. Role sets
  VII. Roles in interaction

Converting Your Topic Outline to a Sentence Outline

For each point in your outline, write one sentence or one definition that
expresses your point of view about that point. As you write out your
definitions, you may find that you will have to revise your outline, since
you may be moving farther away rather than closer to your original
topic. As a handy reminder of your original thinking, you may want to
include an example with your definition. If the definition does not
follow from your example, try to rephrase it so that it says the same
thing to you as the example does.

Role is the set of behaviors that are attached to a particular social position or status within a society.

  I. Role types are the specific roles attached to a particular position within a social position.

    A. Patient role is the set of behaviors expected of individuals who are receiving health care services.

      1. Terminal patient roles are those behaviors expected of patients who are dying.

        a. Those behaviors attached to patients who don't know they are dying, but the staff does know.

        b. Those behaviors attached to patients who do know they are dying.

          1) Terminal patients who have just been told may react with anger, crying, withdrawal, or a request to see their spiritual advisor.

          2) Terminal patients who have known about their diagnosis for some time may be used to the idea, may refuse to talk about it, may talk about their death freely, may be clearing up their personal affairs, may want to be with their families as much as possible.

        c. Those behaviors attached to patients who know they are dying but pretend not to know.

Putting the Theory Back with the Question

By outlining your theory and writing definitions about each relevant aspect, you now have some new working definitions for each term in your question. Not only do you have your terms behaviorally defined, you have also added some new qualifying words to your research question. After your thorough review of role theory, your topic may look more like this:

    cancer patients react to having just been told that they are termi-
    nally ill

In fact, you may have a whole new series of topics based upon your review of theory. But remember, one topic is all you need to do research; more than one makes a very complicated study.

    If you have decided to retain your original question (stem plus topic), you still have to investigate learning theory just as you did with role theory. Remember, in research you will need a working definition of *every* word in your question, and as your question gets longer, you will need to write more definitions. Every word must be moved from the abstract to the particular before you write your problem.

Now that you have asked questions of your theory, defined each term in your question, outlined the relevant aspects of the theory, clarified exactly what you want to observe about each aspect and why, and, finally, substantiated each part of your outline with literature, you have the basic outline of your ideas and your literature review. This outline alone, written in the form of an essay, can easily constitute your theoretical framework for the study. (If you had done the same work on one or more concepts, you would have the underpinnings for a conceptual framework.) If you are dealing with more than one theory or concept, your framework must show their relationship to one another and to your question.

A PROBLEM CLOSE TO HOME

Remember that we began this discussion by saying that starting with a theory and working it down to specific observable phenomena was more difficult than starting with an observation and relating it to specific situations. In the latter instance, you are proceding from your personal experience and familiarity with the subject you are studying.

Suppose you had started with an observation that certain patients reacted differently to learning that they had terminal cancer. Some reacted with anger, shouting, crying, moroseness; others didn't react at all. Your original question might have been:

> What are the differences between oncology patients who react with anger versus those who don't react at all when they are told they are terminally ill?

This question is already observable and measurable. It takes you from the particular situation to the abstract explanation. You may end up explaining the differences by using role theory or you may find an entirely different theory such as stimulus-response or loss theory to explain them. This type of question is easier to write about simply because as a nurse, you are familiar with the subject. You have experienced these behaviors for yourself. You know what you are looking for, and why. And as a nurse, you can probably use the answer in your practice.

Just because you are familiar with your subject and begin with readily observable terms does not mean that you are free from the responsibility of reviewing the literature on your question. On the contrary, because your question is so specific, it may have already been answered by someone else. Your first task, then, is not to look up the theory, but to examine the research literature.

Where do you start?

Just as with the theory question, you begin with each specific idea in your question. In this instance, you will begin with the words *oncology patients*. Card catalogs, the nursing index, and the Index Medicus will have a section on oncology, but may not have anything specific on oncology patients. Just as in the theory question, you must then look up *patients* in the literature. But you are interested in specific patients, those with terminal illnesses, and their reactions to learning about their illnesses. To adequately review the literature on this subject, each aspect of your question needs to be checked out to see who or what has done something that relates specifically or remotely to your question.

As you begin your reading, you will find that certain researchers discuss theories that relate to their research or discuss their findings in relation to new ideas and theories. As you read, take note of these interrelated ideas. One or more of them will strike you as being *the one* concept or theory that truly fits your question.

Just as with the theory question, keep your bibliography cards organized and properly annotated. You will probably want to head your card with the aspect of the question that the reference is talking about, such as *Oncology Patients*. From these cards, an outline will begin to form.

Your outline practically writes itself. Your question is the major heading; your minor headings come from the individual words or specific ideas within the question. This outline takes the reverse of the theory outline format. You will move from your specific definitions to an idea or a concept. For example:

I. Oncology patients are in-patients on an oncology unit who were admitted with a tentative diagnosis of a carcinogenic process.
   A. Diagnostic studies have been completed, diagnosis has been confirmed, patient has been informed that he/she has lung cancer. According to the chart the patient reacted with:
      1. Anger: Explosive and abusive language to the staff and to his/her family.
         a. Anger can be a defense mechanism to protect an individual from an intolerable fact.
         b. Anger can be a normal expression for any disagreeable fact, opinion. Cultural behavior?
         c. Anger can be a usual response for some people. Stimulus/response?
      2. No response: After the patient received his/her diagnosis, chart states that the patient began to make pleasant conversation with the physician, changed the

subject, or otherwise gave no indication that he/she either heard or cared about the diagnosis.

    a. Heard partially. Higher levels of anxiety cause frag-mented (spotty) perceptions.

    b. Denied the meaning of what was heard.

    c. May not wish to discuss the issue until he/she had some time to think about it. Motivation?

    d. May have the behavioral pattern of not discussing intimate details with strangers. Cultural beliefs?

    e. Explanation given may be so vague and technical, patient did not understand.

  B. Diagnostic studies have been completed as in A. Patient has been informed that he/she has leukemia.

  C. Diagnostics as in A and B. Patient informed that he/she has metastatic cancer from prior surgery.

Since there are a variety of reasons for the patient's reactions to diagnosis, and since each type of reaction may have a theoretical explanation, you must decide which theory best fits your question and why the others do not fit.

You established your outline according to your ideas and your reading, but because you began with a behavioral observation, your definition of terms is more specific and more observable at the outset. Your review of research and theory is easier because you know what you are looking for at the beginning.

Starting with a problem close to home gives you the advantage of having more information about your question to start with, which in turn enables you to direct your reading and outline more specifically and to form working definitions.

The second aspect of starting with a problem close to home is that you are usually involved with the question you select. You are either working with the question on a daily basis or have had a recent experi-ence with it that is likely to occur again. For this reason, the work you do on your problem—your thinking, your reading, and your attempts at clarification—is immediately applicable in your daily life and is not just an isolated incident of writing a research proposal. The more removed your research question is from you personally, the more removed you will be in the rest of your project. The more intimately involved you are with your question, the more interest you will generate in yourself, the more likely you are to sustain your interest, and the more practical your work will be.

On the other hand, if working with theory excites you, don't select a problem just because it's practical. Remember, this is your research project and no one else's—so whatever turns you on is the question you need to ask.

RECOMMENDED READING

Campbell, William Giles, and Ballou, Stephen Vaughan. *Form and Style: Theses, Reports, Term Papers.* New York: Houghton Mifflin Co., 1974.

Markman, Roberta H., and Waddell, Marie L. *10 Steps in Writing the Research Paper.* Woodbery, N.Y.: Barron's Educational Series, Inc., 1971.

Menzel, Donald H.; Jones, Howard Mumford; and Boyd, Lyle G. *Writing a Technical Paper.* New York: McGraw-Hill Book Co., 1961.

Strunk, William Jr., and White, E. B. *The Elements of Style.* New York: Mac-Millan Co., 1959.

III.

The Full and Final Problem

Elements of a Research Problem
1. The Rationale for Developing the Question
2. The Theoretical or Conceptual Framework
3. Review of the Literature

The Psychology of Argument
Strongest Argument Last

Substantiating What You Say

Form of the Final Research Problem
1. The Introduction
2. The Body
3. The Conclusion

In learning how to arrive at your full research problem, you developed all the necessary elements for the entire research plan—your question, your theories, your terms defined, and the type of measurement that you intend to use. Your next step is to put all of these components together into a complete package, *the research problem*. This is very much like putting a bicycle together that you ordered from a catalogue. If any of the parts is missing, or if you attached the pedals where the wheels belong, you won't have a workable bicycle. Like the bicycle, the full problem should have a sense of completeness about it; all the parts should operate together, and the problem as a whole should work properly and be aesthetically pleasing. A poorly designed research plan is as useless as a box of parts and bolts.

To extend the analogy: putting a bicycle together is much easier, less time-consuming, and less frustrating if you know the relationship between the parts and of the parts to the whole. If you know the *what* and *why* of the parts to a bicycle, then you know if you are putting things together properly and if you have achieved the full and final bicycle. A well-constructed bicycle is achieved because you know how it works, why it works, and what it needs to work.

A well-constructed research problem is achieved in the same way, because you know how and why it works, and what it needs to work. But before you can build your research problem, you need to understand the basic elements of the problem.

ELEMENTS OF A RESEARCH PROBLEM

Although some research texts and published research papers include all of the introductory matter (problem, rationale, purpose, literature review, and terms) under the heading *Problem*, it's best to know the elements of the problem itself and how it is developed as a separate and distinct section of the research plan. The elements are:

1. The rationale for developing the question
2. The theoretical or conceptual framework
3. The literature review

Each element, for its fullest development, requires a lot of thinking, reorganizing of ideas, and a logical progression of concepts and facts that leads the reader to your statement of purpose. Although research problems can be written in a variety of ways (see the research proposals in the appendix), the same basic elements are present in all problems.

The problem is your frame of reference for the entire research project; your rationale for choice of literature; your point of view on your subject—all of which are substantiated by facts, theories, and arguments gleaned from your reading. The problem is your statement of what you are doing and why. If you are hesitant about your idea, your problem will be hesitant. If you are uninterested in your study, your problem will be dull. If you haven't done your reading, your problem will be merely a "bucket of bolts." Whether you know it or not, your problem is the expression of your personality.

1. *The rationale for developing the question.* The amount of space devoted to the rationale will vary, depending upon the type of question you have chosen to answer. Exploratory studies that do not support the question with research should devote more space to the rationale behind the question than experimental designs that substantiate the question with research findings.

The rationale for asking the question is *your* statement of why you thought of the question, why you want an answer, and of what use the answer will be to nursing. What made you think of the question in the first place? You certainly had a series of ideas or questions that lead you to this final research question. This is your rationale for the development of the question, and if not explicitly stated, must be clear by the time the reader has finished reading the problem argument. This is your logic, your reasoning, your point of view—and the reader has the right to know what it is.

2. *The theoretical or conceptual framework.* Although these words are frightening to the new researcher, they are not as formidable as they sound. A framework is simply the structure of the idea or concept and how it is put together. In this book, we are putting the framework in the form of an *essay,* and the structure of a good essay is in the form of an argument. This essay must support your rationale for developing the question. If the theoretical or conceptual framework contradicts the rationale for developing the question, something is wrong, either in the framework or the question itself, and you had best begin again.

A theoretical framework, then, is an essay that interrelates the theories involved in the question. If your question deals with loss theory or theories of aggression, your theoretical framework should discuss thoroughly the theory (or theories) you are using and show how the theorizing and research lead you to your question and the purpose of your study. The topical outline described in Chapter 2 is the outline of your theoretical framework. If you used more than one theory, you would have to outline and discuss each one separately and then show how they interrelate. In either case, your theoretical framework is simply the theoretical structure for your study.

Conceptual frameworks, like theoretical frameworks, are essays that explain, describe, and analyze all of the ideas inherent in the question in a logical, rational format. If you are not testing a theory, you will need to isolate the major concepts inherent in your question.

And those concepts will need to be discussed in relation to your rationale for developing the question.

Remember, a theory is a discussion of related concepts, while a concept is a word or phrase that symbolizes several interrelated ideas. Unlike a theory, a concept does not need to be discussed to be understood. However, since you are using several interrelated concepts in a new way, your conceptual framework must explain the relationship among these concepts.

Even if your question does not include a theory, there is no doubt that it contains at least one concept that needs to be explained or described in relation to the question as a whole. Look at your question again. How many ideas—as expressed in words—does your question contain? Look at each of your definitions. More than likely it is a sequence of related ideas that form a concept rather than a single idea. If so, you must write a conceptual framework that explains the interrelationship of all of the ideas in your question.

3. *Review of the literature.* The rationale for the development of your question came from somewhere—ideas do not develop in a vacuum. Ideas often come from an outside source, either in written form or in an interview. Your review of the literature simply documents the source of your idea and substantiates the rationale behind your question.

The rationale for incorporating the review of literature in the problem essay, is that when you substantiate what you say, you usually substantiate it through the literature you have read or direct personal quotes. Therefore, since you must document your source for your rationale and your theoretical/conceptual framework—why separate your review of literature from the two other elements in the problem definition? You simply waste paper by repeating your sources in a different way.

The literature review is a series of references, not a bibliography. Only the literature that you have used to substantiate your problem is included in your literature review. Not everything that you have read about your problem is relevant to your research and therefore should not be included in the review. In high school you included your entire bibliography to prove to your teacher that you did extensive reading. But this is research, and only relevant literature is required in the literature review.

When you write your problem essay, you will be incorporating your rationale for the development of the question, your theoretical or conceptual framework, and your literature review into one (not three) definitive statement of what you are studying, and why, and its relevance to you and to your reader.

Remember, at this point you are the expert on your research. Now all that you have to do is prove your expertise in an essay.

THE PSYCHOLOGY OF ARGUMENT

Each element in your research problem is absolutely necessary to persuade the reader that your research project is sound, well thought-out, and well documented from observations or reading. This is the essence of argument—to persuade another person that you are right, to prove beyond a shadow of a doubt that you know what you are talking about, that you are an *authority*.

To argue your point successfully, you will need to know your opposition as well as you know your position. For many of us, that's not an easy thing to do. We are so enamored of our own position we cannot think of any possible argument against it. But notice the technique in successful debates, successful salesmanship, successful books—they have all taken into account the opposition's point of view and had an answer for it. They were prepared to answer any question that required clarification, explanation, or further data. Whether you are trying to entice people to support your organization or accept your research plan, you need to plan ahead to win the argument.

The crux of the matter is, you have stimulated the argument and you are interested in winning. Winning just doesn't happen by itself. So if you are going to start an argument, be prepared to win it. You have the edge, because the opposition is not prepared for an argument nor do they have a vested interest in its outcome.

Let's say that you have already experienced losing your research argument, which went something like this: "I want to study children's reactions to injections." Your instructor looked at you and said, "Well, that sounds like a reasonable enough topic, but why do you want to study it?" Somewhat taken back by being questioned at all, you respond with, "I'm in pediatrics and I think it would be good to know." A pained expression comes over your instructor's face, perhaps even a sigh, and all of a sudden you feel pretty inadequate.

Suppose you had said instead, "I'm on a peds ward and I've noticed differences in children's reactions to injections. I have a hunch that there is a difference in boys' and girls' reactions after, say, about the age of five because of the way children are socialized into sexually stereotyped role reactions to painful experiences. I'm not sure just when—what age, I mean—these differences begin to be noticed, nor am I sure if it has anything to do with previous experiences with injections. But it seems to me that if we could find out when those differences occur—if they do, and if there is any relationship between prior experience, age, and sex, we as nurses could then change our approach to giving children medications on the basis of these findings."

Result? Full approval and a go-ahead.

Why? Because you thought out your rationale for why you want to do your study, you gave a personal observation to back up your idea, you suggested a theory to explain your observation, and you pointed out a use for the information that you might gather from your study. You won your argument simply because you answered all of the questions. Your position was logical, sound, and thoughtful. Perhaps without knowing it, you incorporated all of the elements on problem selection. You spoke with authority.

Your argument also had a basic structure. You began with the general problem area that you wanted to study. Then you conceded that you don't know all the answers ("I have a hunch . . ."), and third, you pointed out the practicality of the project. This was your punch line, which you shrewdly left for the end. Strong arguments always include 1) central points, 2) concessions, and 3) the points in favor of the position.

The basic elements of the full problem follow the requirements for an argument. Your rationale for developing the question uses the style of argument—the central issue you are dealing with, the many and diverse ideas or situations that could be explored through research, and your reason for settling on this particular project. Your argument is strengthened by your literature review. Each point you make in a concession, or in your favor, should have relevant, documented facts to substantiate your statements.

The conceptual or theoretical framework also follows the logic of argument, whether you integrate your framework into your rationale for developing the question, or write it as a separate section. You will begin with your central point, make concessions to other relevant theories or concepts, and then point out exactly which theory or concept is most applicable to your study and why. Here again, your literature review substantiates your basic framework.

Whether you are doing research on a theory, an observation, or a particular tool, use the psychology of argument in the development of your problem.

Strongest Argument Last

Imagine for a moment that you are the teacher of a research course, and all of your students had handed in their problems for you to read. Which of the following problems would you make the student rewrite and which would convince you?

Problem 1: Recently-bereaved widows have greater difficulties adjusting to the social problems of daily living than the literature on bereavement suggests. Most of the research and theory in bereavement deals with the phenomena of psychological adjustments to loss. Nurses need to know more about loss and grief. This study will add to the body of knowledge on loss and grief in widows.

Problem 2: Nurses are constantly interacting with patients who have suffered some form of loss, the death of a spouse or child, loss of a job, or loss of a limb. Most theories on loss are psychological explanations in relation to grief or bereavement. Few studies have explored the relationship between a particular loss and the resulting daily social adjustments that must be made. Yet a major area of nursing care is to assist the patient with problems of daily living and adjustment to the loss—not just to assist patients to cope psychologically without the lost object. Therefore, a study that focuses on the social adjustments to loss should provide nurses with some ways to assist the patient in adjusting to the social changes resulting from the loss. For this reason, this study will focus on the social adjustments of daily living that newly bereaved widows must make.

If you agree that Problem 2 made the strongest statement, look at the structure of the problem again. Notice that it begins with a generalization and ends with a specific, from loss to widows' daily adjustments to a loss. Then it builds to a climax, "Therefore, a study which focuses on . . .," and presents the final, irrefutable argument supporting the focus of this study. Finally, the problem deals with the usefulness of the data to be learned. The structure of the argument is maintained by listing concessions first and points in favor later. The movement in Problem 2 is from the problem area to the purpose of the study. In one paragraph, the skeletal outline for the entire research problem has been presented.

On the other hand, Problem 1 starts with the specific and ends with a generality; it made the major point first and ended on a weak note. The same argument is presented in Problem 1 as in Problem 2, but the ordering of the problem is different. Putting the strongest argument last leaves a stronger impression in the mind of the reader, who will have forgotten the first sentence by the end of the paragraph. The last sentence is the one the reader will remember; therefore, it should be the strongest.

Notice that Problem 2 is longer than Problem 1, even though they are both single paragraphs. This is due to the logic of the argument. When you begin your argument with your major point, it is difficult to create concessions and defenses afterwards. If you start with the general problem, make concession, and then build your defense from minor to major points, your argument is necessarily longer. But because of its structure, you can easily check it to see that you haven't left anything out.

Read a good essay, article, or research report, and notice the way the author leads you from the general to the specific, from minor to major points, from concessions to defense. Remember that the advantage is always to the person who has the final, definitive argument.

SUBSTANTIATING WHAT YOU SAY

By this point, you should have in your research workbook your research question; your topical outline of your theories, concepts or observations; your working definitions of every major term in your question; and a one-paragraph statement of your entire problem area. In other words, you should have the skeleton for the final research problem for your written proposal. Before you proceed to write the full and final problem as an essay, you have one final area to check— your review of literature, since it is this that substantiates your argument.

Look at Problem 2 again. Notice the sentences that begin: "Most theories on loss . . ." and "Few studies . . ." In your full and final problem, you can't get away with those statements just as they are. You have to justify those statements with facts. Here is where your review of the literature comes in.

To be at this stage in your project where you have the skeleton for your final problem, you had to have done some reading. If you have bibliography cards or annotated references on everything you have read, you are now ready to build a case for your project.

Begin the process with your research question, which is, after all, the central point you are trying to make. Put it up somewhere in front of you so that you can refer to it frequently. Now reread your question. Which is the most central point you are trying to make in your question? Which is the topic of the question, the major thrust around which all the rest of the question revolves? Underline that portion of the question. Take every other word or phrase and rank them under the central point in descending order of importance. Do your outline and definitions agree with this order? If not, look at your question again. Does it include your strongest argument? If not, you need to rewrite it. Your question must contain your strongest argument.

Now take your outline and arrange each point under the headings you made from your question. You are now restructuring your outline from the most relevant issues to the least relevant. You also have a reference for each point in your outline. Separate the pros and cons under each heading. Make sure that for each heading you have references both in favor of and against that point.

As you work with your question and your outline, you will begin to notice two things happening to your notes. One, you will find interesting but irrelevant pieces of information. Set those aside. You may need them later, but right now you are building your argument and you don't need them. Second, you may find that some of your notes fit under more than one topic heading. That always happens. Cross-reference your topic headings so that you can easily find your notes. Sometimes a reading will give both the pros and cons for the subject. Don't throw them out. You can always use the same author or even the same reading in several different places.

You now have a topic outline of your problem from the strongest to weakest argument with concessions and defense. And for each topic heading, you have a list of readings. Recheck your outline to see if there are any gaps in your argument. Does every heading in your outline have at least two contrasting subcategories? Does your argument include both pros and cons? Do you feel you are an authority? Are you confident that you can defend your position from any point of view?

If you feel that you are being overwhelmed with reams and reams of paper, there is another way of developing the outline for your problem. Outline the central and substantiating areas of your question. Then arrange your annotated cards under the appropriate outline headings. Now arrange each group of cards according to the major and minor points. Then divide the cards under each heading according to pros and cons. Instead of a written outline, you now have your reference cards sorted into an outline. This is the advantage of writing references on 5 × 8 cards. They are easier to sort and they hold up better than paper.

You might want to use a shoe box or a card file and make dividers under each content heading to keep your cards sorted. That way, as you begin your problem essay, all you have to do is pull out the appropriate cards and write directly from them. This method saves wear-and-tear on your nerves and prevents the loss of that one significant point you want to make.

The critical point in this discussion is that you have ready references for every point you are making in your problem. You can quickly and easily substantiate your position with a quote, a paraphrase, or a reference to authors who have said essentially the same thing. Because you have done your homework, you can prove your point—you have become an authority.

FORM OF THE FINAL RESEARCH PROBLEM

Whether you end up with one page or twenty-one, the full and final research problem has the same form and shape. Like an essay, article, or term paper, the research problem has an introduction, a middle, and a conclusion. In fact, your final problem has the same requirements as a good essay—you introduce your question, you point out the pros and cons for your argument, and you end with the statement of what you are going to study and why. The rest of the research plan is an expansion, an explication of your problem.

Your research plan is only as good as your research problem. If you have a strong method but a weak problem, you will have a weak piece of research. Although the reverse is just as true, it's easier to salvage a weak method than a weak problem. There is nothing worse than using a sophisticated method to answer a trifling problem. Even if anyone reads it, few will use it, and all your work is wasted. And since usability is a keynote for research, you don't want your efforts considered irrelevant. So, for now, concentrate on writing the best possible problem. Not only will you have a sense of satisfaction, your credibility level will go up enormously.

The Introduction

Regardless of the length of your problem, you must introduce your topic to your reader. All introductions follow the same pattern and include the same kinds of information. Your introduction does not need to be any longer than one paragraph—and a short one at that— but if it isn't there, it's like being pushed into a swimming pool with all your clothes on. The introduction is the preparation for the rest of your discussion.

Introductions are exactly what you think they are: they introduce the subject under discussion.

The first sentence in the introduction sets the *general* tone and direction for the subject matter. The middle sentence or sentences narrows the focus. The last sentence is your research question written as a statement, and begins with such words as *therefore, in conclusion,* or *finally.* You are moving your reader from the general to the specific.

The first sentence of your introduction can be an observation, a quote, a paraphrase, or a question. But its major function is to present the subject, interest the reader, and start the ball rolling. You may have to rewrite it several times to get the feel of a good first sentence. Or you may want to start with the middle and write the first sentence later. Either way that suits your style is fine; just don't forget to include the first sentence in your final introduction.

What is the general subject area you intend to pursue? Are you introducing your reader to loss, denial, surgical patients or a specific attitude? Say so. Don't mince around. If you keep your readers guessing, they lose interest quickly. Establishing interest is important, even if it is only your teacher who will be reading your work.

On the other hand, a first sentence filled with exclamation points can be just as uninteresting. Let your reader fill in the exclamation points for you. Your object is to be clear, precise, and to the point.

Write your sentence from any of the major nouns in your question. Make sure that your first sentence is general, or at least more general than your question. Don't present your argument or your position, just introduce the idea. Your last sentence states your position, so save the punch line for it.

Your next sentences follow the logic of argument, as we have already discussed. Make your concessions to other points of view—but make them brief. Use the concessions to narrow your focus. Sometimes one sentence will do, at other times two or more will be necessary. This depends entirely on the complexity of your problem. Look again at Problem 2 in the *Strongest Argument Last* section. This problem could easily substitute for an introductory paragraph. The middle sentences would have to be reworded somewhat to meet the criteria of the opening paragraph. Instead of saying, "most theories on loss . . .," you would hedge more. You would say something like, "Some theories on loss . . ." The next sentence would lead off with something like, "Other studies have explored . . ."

The middle sentences narrow the topic down, giving some detail on what is to come next. But still don't hit the reader with the full and final argument.

The last sentence in your introduction is your reworded question. The last sentence ties up with the first sentence and gives a feeling of unity to the introduction. The opening phrases (*therefore, for this reason,* and *finally*) all tell the reader that this is the one central point you will deal with.

The purpose of writing a research question at the beginning is becoming clearer.

One further function of the introductory paragraph is that it tells the reader, and yourself as well, what the rest of the research problem will discuss; it is the abstract of your problem. The rest of the problem is an expansion of your introductory paragraph, in which each sentence will be substantiated, argued, and proven.

The Body

The body of the problem is where you present arguments for and against your project. You can subtitle your problem according to the concepts you are discussing, or you can have one long uninterrupted series of arguments from general to specific. Whether you use sub-heads or not is up to you. But use the psychology of argument here. Start with the weakest part of your argument and build up to your major point. Also be sure that you account for the three major elements of the problem: rationale, literature review, and theoretical/conceptual framework.

Use your theory or concept outline and your references here. Fill in the outline with your reading. Paraphrase as much as possible. There is nothing more boring than reading a series of quotes. The reader wants to know what *you* think, what *your* argument is; if they want other opinions, they can check the sources you have cited. So write this section in your own words as much as possible. When you absolutely cannot improve or paraphrase an author's statement, then quote, but only sparingly.

Use repetition only for emphasis. If you want to emphasize a point, paraphrase several authors making the same statement. Or quote one, paraphrase another, and list several others who have said essentially the same thing. But use this technique only to emphasize major points. Otherwise, quote or paraphrase the originator of an idea or research and then simply list the authors who agree. You can type pages and pages of everyone's position on the same idea, but all that work goes unread and does not save our trees.

Since you are using your references to substantiate your points, you may find yourself beginning each statement with "Jones said," or "Maxwell stated," or "According to Pinchpenny." Don't worry about it as you are working on the body of your problem. But *never, never* let it stand that way. After you have finished writing the body, and have exhausted every single argument for and against each and every part of your question, go back and rewrite every sentence that begins with "Jones stated," or "A comment by Jones et al." Reference Jones at the end of the quote or at the end of your paraphrased paragraph. The whole point in the body of your problem is to maintain the flow of ideas, not to list sources. When you introduce each sentence with a source, you are essentially writing a who's who in the literature, not a statement of your argument. And the difference is critical.

As you develop the body of your problem, remember to leave the strongest, most central point for the last. Since you are leading your reader along the path of your logic, you want to make your strongest point just before your conclusion. You want to leave the impression that there is not one single *i* that has not been dotted, a single comma left out, or a point neglected. You have used and manipulated each and every outline to its fullest extent and you have lead up to your research question—again.

The Conclusion

Like the introduction, the conclusion should be no more than one paragraph in length. Unlike an essay, in which the conclusion moves from the specific back to the general for closure, the conclusion of the research problem serves as the introduction to the rest of the research plan. Your conclusion pulls all the strands of your argument together and ties up any loose ends. It ends with your research question, written either in the form of a question, if it fits the style of your preceding sentences, or as a statement. Usually your question is better rewritten as a statement introduced by "Therefore, this study . . ." or "For this reason, this study . . ." or "As a result, this study . . ."

Your conclusion places your rationale, your thinking, and your arguments into one neat package. You want to leave the reader—and yourself—with the feeling that there is nothing further to be said, explained, or argued about your choice of topic. You have closed the door on this aspect of your proposal.

One way of writing a conclusion is to rephrase the introduction. Since the body of the problem simply expanded and explained the introduction, the conclusion can restate the introduction with authority. In this way, the conclusion ties in with both the introduction and the problem, and the sense of completeness is achieved.

At the same time, the conclusion also leaves the reader on a high note, a sense of anticipation of what is to come. This is achieved through the restatement of the research question that appeared in the introduction. Although this brings the reader full circle from question back to question, the answer and how it is to be achieved are yet to come. And the reader is fully aware of this if your problem is well written.

So, keeping in mind that you don't need to repeat everything you have already said, use your conclusion to pull together all of the major points covered in the body of the problem and lead directly into the research question. Remember: keep it brief, keep it to the point, and keep it interesting. The reader now knows the best is yet to come.

RECOMMENDED READING

Chater, Shirley. "Search or Research? The Teaching of Selecting and Stating the Problem." *Nursing Outlook* 13 (1965): 65.

Diers, Donna. "Finding Clinical Problems for Study." *Journal of Nursing Administration*, November–December 1971, pp. 15–18.

Vaughn, Lucille Payne. *The Lively Art of Writing.* Philadelphia: Mentor Books, 1965.

Wandelt, Mabel. *Guide for the Beginning Researcher.* New York; Appleton-Century-Crofts, 1970.

IV.

The Structure of the Research Proposal

The Introductory Matter
1. The Problem
2. Purpose and Hypothesis
3. Definition of Terms

The Research Design
1. Introduction
2. The Sample
3. Methods and Instruments
4. Reliability and Validity
5. Analysis of Data

Protection of Human Rights

There are two major parts to any research plan, whether you write it for yourself, a class, or a grant proposal: the *introductory matter* and the *research design*. Both parts are always present, though the titles may differ. Each part has its particular components, though they too may have different terms. Both the structure and the components within the structure are derived from the research question.

Chapters I, II, and III described the process of converting the topic of your research question into the *problem* of the research proposal. Since the research question is the basis for your research plan, and since the problem is the foundation of the rest of the research proposal, the emphasis on these two areas was quite deliberate.

Your research question is your guide to what you have to do and think and read and plan in order to arrive at your research proposal. Your question is an activity guide; your proposal is the end product. Put another way, your question is process; your proposal is content.

The difference between question and proposal is the same difference you found in planning patient assessment and the actual assessment in the Nursing Care Plan. When you plan your assessment, you begin by gathering information from the patient, the patient's chart, textbooks on the pathology and medical intervention, and by looking up medications and treatments with which you are not familiar. You then put all of this data together, analyze it, and arrive at your final formulation of the patient's problems and needs. The culmination of all your questioning, reading, and analysis is written in a final form called an Assessment. You didn't write down your entire step-by-step process; you wrote only the end result.

The same process is used for the research proposal. The question guides and directs your activities; the proposal is your end result.

Since the basic structure and the components of the research plan are fairly standardized, and since each component is based on the previous ones, we are going to discuss each of the basic components in turn. In addition, the concepts of reliability and validity of the research and the protection of human rights for the people involved will also be discussed even though their placement in the proposal is not as standardized. Omitting them from the proposal would seriously jeopardize your chances of eventually doing your project.

THE INTRODUCTORY MATTER

You will rarely see the title *The Introductory Matter* in any research report or proposal. Usually the titles are *Introduction, Rationale, Conceptual* or *Theoretical Framework,* or even *What This Study Is All About.* Whatever the title, the purpose of the first section is to introduce the reader to the subject matter of the research. This introduction should always include the *problem,* the *purpose* or *hypotheses,* and *definitions of terms.* The order may vary, but not the content.

The Problem. The first portion of any proposal introduces the subject matter of the research, the rationale for selecting the problem, the literature to substantiate the rationale, and the direction the study will take. As you have seen, the problem derives from the topic of the research question. Some problems are a paragraph long, others a full chapter, still others may take two or three chapters, one to cover the theoretical or conceptual framework, another to review the literature, and still another for the historical development of the idea. If you have thought through your problem well, the theory and the literature will substantiate your choice of topic. You don't need to be repetitive to put your point across. You can, however, sub-head your problem according to the different theories or concepts that relate to your subject. But a well written problem should introduce the entire research plan under the one heading.

Purpose and Hypotheses. Remember from Chapter III that the end of the problem is a lead-in to the specific study, which is the research question. If you have written your problem well, you don't have to again introduce your question or explain why you are asking it. Instead, your question is a separate entity; your problem merely leads the reader to it.

But you ask, "Why call it a purpose or a hypothesis if I am asking a question?" Chapter VI goes into more detail on the answer to that question, but briefly, let's put it this way.

The purpose of all research is to answer the question. So under the heading *Purpose* you would say: "The purpose of this study is to answer the question . . ." Or you could transpose your question into a declarative statement and say: "The purpose of this study is to . . ." and write your question as a statement. Hypotheses, which you have encountered in the literature, are simply the if-then form of the question.

The criteria for deciding when to use a question, a declarative statement, or a hypothesis is discussed in Chapter VI. Just remember that the purpose of the study is to answer the question, no matter in what form it is written.

You now have the basis for your entire research proposal—the research problem and the purpose of your study. All the rest of the proposal is an expansion and clarification of those two areas.

Definition of Terms. The next step is to provide the reader with your *operational* definitions of each term used in your purpose. You must show how you intend to measure or evaluate each aspect of your question. You may have to re-write your working definitions after doing the reading, but the point is that *every* term—whether it's your sample, your subject, your theory, or your observation—must be clearly spelled out in relation to: 1) *what* specifically you intend to study; and 2) *how* you intend to study or measure it. Defining terms is an inescapable fact in the life of the researcher.

Although you were introduced to working definitions in Chapter I, a full discussion of changing *working* definitions to *operational* definitions is provided in Chapter VII.

You have now finished all of the introductory matter in your proposal. You have introduced your research subject and explained the reasons for your choice; you have explained who you are studying, the theoretical basis for your study, and how you will measure your terms. You are now ready to proceed to the research design.

THE RESEARCH DESIGN

You may have noticed in reading the table of contents that the chapter on research design is subtitled, "Blueprint for Action." That's exactly what the design is all about. It is your blueprint, or guide, to your activity. If you have ever seen the blueprint or plan of a house, you know that on one page is a master print of the building, which gives the number of stories and their basic outlines. You can see the number of rooms on each floor, the relationship of the rooms to one another, the placement of doors and windows, and so on. Succeeding pages deal with each room separately. The smaller the area being planned, the more specific the detail. Your research design follows the same principle. Your introductory material is your master plan; you are now going to deal with each section separately and in detail.

Introduction.　Although not required, it is often helpful to introduce the design with a general statement about what it will encompass. Frequently this introduction states the general direction the research will take: exploratory, descriptive, explanatory, or experimental. This puts the reader in the right frame of reference, and also makes you more careful in handling the rest of your proposal.

The Sample.　Although you have introduced your sample under the definition of terms—who you intend to include and exclude from your particular population—you must now describe in detail how you intend to make your selection, how many people will be in your sample, where you will find them and how you intend to approach them, what you intend to do if you have dropouts or no-shows, and so forth.

To be sure your sample indeed represents your population, you will need some hard facts from the literature for verification. You will need to describe the demographic characteristics of your sample—age, sex, educational level, occupation, religion—because they will affect analysis as well as data collection.

Methods and Instruments. You should now describe the method(s) you intend to use to collect your data. These might include anything from questionnaires and interviews to projective tests or laboratory experiments. If you are using more than one method, you will need to explain your rationale for each method, how they interrelate and why they are appropriate in view of your sample selection. (See Chapter XI.)

Your methods must be consistent with your sample.

On the basis of the method(s) you have selected, you are now ready to discuss which research instrument you have chosen to collect the data from your sample. You will need to explain why you chose this instrument over others, discuss its strengths and weakness, and outline what tests of reliability and validity have been done on the instrument and on what populations it has been used before. If you have decided to develop your own instrument, the same type of rationale must be presented. Always keep in mind that *the instruments must be consistent with the methods.*

Here again, just as with the sample and the methods, you will need to have reviewed the literature thoroughly in order to present your arguments for your choice of instrument with an authoritative voice.

Reliability and Validity. Although the concepts of reliability and validity can be incorporated into the discussion of the research instrument, they are important enough to deserve a separate section. For one thing, reliability and validity do not apply just to research instruments alone; they are also applicable in analysis of data. So to call attention to the fact that they are an integral part of the proposal, they are given a discussion section of their own. (See Chapter XII.)

Analysis of Data. Many beginners wonder how they can possibly plan to analyze data without some data to analyze. And so they generally ask if they should "make up" some data and analyze it. In a way, they are quite right. "Making up" data is simply a concrete form of projecting what answers you hope to get from the responses to your question. So if you would feel more comfortable projecting or thinking up some data to analyze, go right ahead. The same principles apply in the data analysis plan as in the previous steps of planning.

Your data analysis is the direct product of the information you hope to collect from your sample with data collection instrument. So your plan for data analysis is the projection of your sample data with your method and your instrument. You will begin by categorizing your sample and the information from your instrument. By putting the two sets of categories together, you will develop new categories of answers. Depending upon your sample, method and instrument, you can verbally describe your data, plot on a chart or graph what you found, subject it to descriptive statistics (means, medians and modes), or evolve a plan for inferential statistics.

Because planning ahead for data analysis can be the biggest stumbling block for the novice, an entire chapter has been devoted to this particular portion of the proposal. (See Chapter XIII.) Without an adequate data analysis plan, a perfectly splendid proposal will fall flat on its face.

Just remember, no matter what you plan to do, *the data analysis plan must be consistent with the sample and the instruments.*

You have now completed the basic outline for the research design section of the proposal. And you noticed that each section followed directly from the previous ones. Over and over you read, *this must be consistent with that.* Since each section is based on the previous ones, they must be logically related. But you must show this relationship. You must make the connection; close any gaps. In other words, don't drop bombs! Don't throw something into a section because it looks sophisticated. If it doesn't fit, don't use it. If it wasn't introduced, it doesn't belong.

And finally, you will have noticed that periodically a reference was made to looking something up in the literature. Just insert that statement in each and every aspect of the proposal. You weren't really finished with your literature review when you wrote your problem. Every item in your proposal demands the voice of authority. If you don't know anything about reliability and validity, look it up. If you don't know which method of data analysis to use, look it up. If you don't know anything about your sample or your methods, go to the literature. No one else can do this for you. Since you have to have a rationale for every part of the proposal, make sure your rationale is based on fact, not hearsay. By the end of your proposal you are not just an expert in your content area, you are an expert on the people you are studying, a particular method and design, and a specific form of data analysis. And by becoming an expert you have developed more credibility. You will be sought out by your peers and by employers because of your expertise. And you will have developed self-confidence in yourself as a nurse researcher.

PROTECTION OF HUMAN RIGHTS

When you write up your research proposal in its final form, you have the option of putting your statement on the protection of human rights at the end of the proposal in a section of its own or in the *Sample* section. Either place is perfectly appropriate.

Chapter XIV discusses this section of the proposal in greater detail with an emphasis on the legal requirements. You need to be reminded of human rights here, because your proposal will not be viable if your choice of sample and your data collection methods violate human rights.

As you work on your proposal, keep in mind that your sample has the right to know what they are getting into when they agree to be part of your study. Deliberately misleading your sample to get data is a thing of the past. You must tell them the area of your study, the possible risks if they participate, and what benefits and protection will be available to them. If you can't get permission directly from your sample, you must get permission from the responsible authorities. If you are using available data, the person in charge of that data will need to know the purpose for which you are using it. The person or persons with the right and responsibility to give permission is the one to be approached —whether that person is a member of the sample or responsible for it.

So as you plan your research, remember that straightforward, honest techniques of data collection are more likely to be approved by a committee for the protection of human rights than a piece of research based on eavesdropping, deliberate distortions, or falsification of information to the subjects.

Think of it this way: You may be a member of a research sample someday. How would *you* like to be treated?

V.

Critical Review of the Literature

Whether you have been reading extensively or just enough to get by, the nature of the material and your approach to it make the difference between a simple reading and a *critical* review of the literature. The term *critical review* does not imply criticism, although that can happen. A critical review means taking an *analytical* approach to your reading. When you read critically, you are analyzing what you are reading.

An analytical approach to any literature review implies *purposive* reading. You are reading the literature for a particular purpose. You want some information on a particular subject that you can use. So the first criterion for the critical review is *usability*, just as with research itself. Whether you plan to use the material for general background information or as a reference in your proposal, whether it is a research report or theoretical, your purpose for reading is practical.

Many people have less trouble deciding on the usability of theory. The theory "felt right" or explained something not fully understood. On the other hand, the usability of a research report is not as readily perceived. The findings may have supported your hypothesis, but whether or not you could use the report depends on your ability to understand the report and its conclusions. In order to use research, you have to know what the author is talking about.

Some people feel immediately defeated when they are asked to read research. They say, "I just don't understand statistics." But look again at the structure of the research plan—how much of the plan is statistical? Very, very little. The structure of the research report is exactly the same as the research plan, except that the report is written in past tense. So don't feel frightened by the statistics; that's only one part of research and you can get some help with it if you have understood the rest of the report.

Someone else will sigh and say, "But I just don't have a logical mind, so there's no point in my reading research." Nonsense. Very few people are completely illogical. You may think differently from other people, but this doesn't make you illogical. Did it ever occur to you that perhaps the reason why you couldn't understand the report was because the report was illogical? It's possible, you know. Just because a piece of research is published doesn't mean it's good research or even well written. So don't decide you can't understand research until you've had a chance to evaluate the reports yourself.

Evaluating a research report for its usability is a simple matter of asking a series of questions about the report. The answers to your questions will give you an index of usability.

The second criterion for any research critique is *completeness*. When you read research, you need to be reasonably certain that the report is comprehensive, that it answers all of your questions about a particular topic area—the problem, the sample, the data collection technique, and how the data was analyzed. As you read, are you still left with some questions? Do you feel that you don't quite understand the point being made? If so, the author probably left something out.

A good way to check for completeness is to see the basis of the information given in the report, if you can *replicate* the study. If you have to ask the author for more information before you can do the study, the report is incomplete.

Incomplete studies are very easy to spot. Look for the key words in the research: *purpose, problem, hypotheses, definitions, sample, methods, analysis*. Does the author give you complete information on each area? Or are there omissions, such as who forms the sample—the author giving only who is excluded. Does the author forget to tell you about the interview if one was used? These and other gaps mean you cannot use the report as the basis for a similar research project, so its usability index goes down.

The third criterion is *consistency*. Every area of the report must proceed logically from the previous ones. Can you follow the logical progression of ideas from problem, to purpose, sample, data collection, analysis, and, finally, conclusions? Does the sample section follow from the problem? Is the data analysis consistent with the sample? Or were some of the research subjects thrown out without explanation? Whether you start with the conclusions and recommendations and read back or begin with the introductory matter, the relationship between each component of the research process needs to be clear and logical. If the report is inconsistent, it is incomplete and therefore not usable.

Your review of the literature, therefore, is your analysis of its usability, completeness, and consistency. In your best judgment, and according to your own logic, *you* decide if what you have read will serve your purpose.

A final point needs to be made. Don't expect perfection! Not everyone is perfect—not even published researchers. So don't "throw the baby out with the bathwater" when you are reading research. Evaluate the report with a critical eye. Look for ideas you can use— even a poor report might offer something useful. Look for ways of improving on the research.

CONTENT OF A CRITIQUE

Despite everything you may have heard, read, or thought before, the purpose of a research critique is to find out if the findings are usable for *you*. Since you are the person who is doing the reading, and since you are the person who needs to know if you can use the research, you need to know how to find out if you can use it.

You may have noticed in your reading that some journals regularly publish a critical review or a critique along with the published research. These critiques are done by professionals who know research forward and backward. They bring up points and issues that other people may not have thought of; their critique is as thorough and as detailed as time and space allow. These types of critiques have specific purposes: 1) they raise points that should be considered in further research on the problem, 2) they provide an analysis of the entire research process for people who don't know how to critique, and 3) they add information about one or more aspects of the research process that can be used by other researchers.

As a beginner, you are not expected to do such an extensive critique. But if you look over these critiques, you will observe that the same general questions are asked, and in the same order, as those discussed in the following pages. Only the detail is missing.

WHAT TO CRITIQUE

Unless a critique has already been presented in conjunction with a research report, you will be expected to critique every piece of research literature you read. Remember that you must be able to supply reasons for your choice of material and the way you use it in your proposal. Your critique should supply you with these reasons. No matter which aspect of your project you are attempting to substantiate with the literature, you will need a rationale for inclusion or exclusion of the relevant material. And your rationale is always based upon your analysis of the literature.

Remember, all research is subject to a critique, including yours. The best research has been critiqued from the inception of the idea all the way through to the published report. But until you, the reader, have critiqued the report yourself, you have no way of knowing if it is, in fact, good research.

With this in mind, let's move on to the actual technique of doing a research critique.

HOW TO DO A CRITIQUE

There are several methods of doing a critique; which one you choose depends on your background and experience. The more experienced you become in critiquing and the more you know about research, the more detailed you will become in your analysis. But when you are starting out, you simply need some basic guidelines to follow. You will be surprised at how good you become at critiquing as you go along.

Before you critique an article, even before you read the paper all the way through, scan the conclusions and recommendations. Using your usability index, decide if you want to read the rest of the paper. If you can't use the findings or recommendations, you probably won't want to use the rest of the report, either. If you are looking for a particular research instrument, scan the section on methods or design to see if it is there. If you can't use the material, you will not be interested enough in the full report to critically analyze its contents. So before you commit yourself to an article, scan it for usability and interest.

After selecting an article for your critique, scan the entire article from beginning to end. Look for the key terms listed in Chapter IV: *problem, purpose, terms, design, methods, findings, analysis, protection of human rights,* and *conclusions.* Is each area of the report given a sub-heading that corresponds with each step in the research process? They usually aren't, in which case you should reread the report and under-line each of the major topic headings. (Of course, you do this on your own Xerox copy of the article, not in the journal itself.) If you cannot find a title to underline, then jot your own key term in the margin. This way you give yourself an easy reference guide to all of the steps in the process.

Now scan the order of the headings. Do they follow the ordering you have learned? For example, can you find the introductory matter in the headings or are they somewhere else? Whether you had to label the content yourself or the author provided the appropriate headings, you are looking for the logical progression of the material in the report.

You now have a basic outline of the report's content. Now look for basic gaps. Has any area been left out? Make a note of that to yourself. You may have missed it in your scan, or it may not be there. In either case, you will be looking for gaps and misplaced material as you continue your critique.

Now go back to the article and look at the section you have labeled as either Introduction or the Problem. Read that section carefully and watch for three things: *clarity, significance,* and *documentation.* You will decide on the basis of these three items if the report is substandard, defective or adequate.

A defective problem lacks clarity, significance, and documen-tation of earlier work. The writing style is ambiguous, unclear (you don't know the point being made), and inconsistent. The research itself is either meaningless, unsolvable, or trivial. Either the documentation is missing entirely or the references are incorrect.

A substandard problem is *either* incomplete or unclear, is of limited interest, or is not fully documented.

An adequate or standard problem on the other hand, covers all of the major research objectives. The writing style is clear—you know and understand what the research is about—and the progression of ideas is logical. The documentation of the problem seems to be reasonably complete and used correctly. Finally, its significance is clear in that the problem needed solving or the results are immediately usable.

In order to make this evaluation of the problem, you first have to identify it. If the author doesn't clearly label it, you must find it on your own, which means reading the report thoroughly. Use your outline of the article as your guide. If you find yourself reading about the sample or data collection, you are beyond the problem. Go back to the introduction and look for the problem there. It might be stated as a question, a statement, or a hypothesis. You decide how well or how badly it's stated—but first you have to determine what it is.

Just as with the problem, your analysis of the research design will be based upon your evaluation of the report as either defective, substandard, or adequate. You will be looking at the sample, the methods of data collection, and the analysis.

A defective sample is one that is too limited for the population being studied because it does not represent the population in a logical manner. The sample may have nothing to do with the population. Or it may not be fully described in the article—you really don't know anything about the sample after you read about it. You may feel that the author selected a biased sample from the population. If the sample is meaningless, inconsistent with the problem, or biased, it is defective.

A substandard sample is not quite so bad. The author is either clear as to the population and not the sample or clear as to the sample but not the population it represents. You may find the sample meaningful to the problem but not to the population. Or you might have a hunch that something is wrong within the sample but you're not sure what.

An adequate sample is clearly specified and defined, and clearly related to the particular population and problem being studied. It is representative.

As you recall, data collection methods are based upon the problem and the sample. Again you will be looking for the clarity, significance, and documentation of the methods in relation to the adequacy of the report.

If the data collection methods have no relationship to either the problem or the sample, or if they are simply not presented, they are defective. Phrases like "an interview was conducted," "a questionnaire was constructed," "available data were used," unqualified by further information, are insufficient. Remember, if you cannot use the information—if you cannot replicate the research on the basis of the information given—the study is defective.

Substandard methods give only partial information. You may have a general idea of what the author has done, but not enough detail to use the information. If the author used a reference for the method, go to that reference and look it up. If the reference is unavailable to you from the usual sources and you have to write the author to get the reference, the report is inadequate. On the other hand, you may have full and complete information on the methods used, but you decide on the basis of your reading that only a partial or tentative solution can be achieved through this method.

An adequate or standard report on methods will tell you what was done, and why and how it was done in sufficient detail that you are satisfied that you know enough about the methods to make an informed decision about it.

Remember that the method must be logically consistent with the problem and the sample. Look at the age of the report you are reading. Is it an old piece of research? Was there any work done in that area prior to the time this research was conducted? If not, the relationship between problem, sample, and method is critical. If the work is new, does the author rely on prior literature to establish the relationship between problem, sample and methods? Or does the article deviate completely from established sequences? When the methods are irrelevant to the problem, the research is illogical and defective.

At this point in your critiquing career, your analysis of data is rough and somewhat skimpy. Unless you know statistics inside and out, you will have some difficulties with this part of the critique. Nevertheless, you should have some idea of what to look for. Again, you are looking at the clarity of the reporting style, the documentation of method, and the relationship between analysis and method.

Most research reports have tables of information, charts, and graphs. Can you find the sample adequately represented in the table? What about the methods—are they exemplified anywhere? If you were to block out an answer to the question based on the methods and sample, what would you include? Look to see if the author has included this critical information.

A defective analysis does not answer the question that was asked. Such an analysis is unclear, ambiguous, unrelated to the data, or inconsistent with the rest of the research. A substandard analysis shows bias toward one aspect of the data over another, or does not fully present an analytical tool. The adequate analysis on the other hand, is comprehensible, responsive to the data, and congruent with all preceding material in the article.

Finally you are ready to examine that aspect of the report that discusses findings, conclusions, and usability of the research. You have read the report quite thoroughly to this point and can form an impression of the findings or conclusions. Are they unclear? Ambiguous? Irrelevant to the preceding material? Unusable?

The findings and conclusions do have to be generated from the research. If the researcher makes some assumptions or conclusions that have not been adequately substantiated elsewhere in the report, you may suspect bias. One small research project, as you know, will not solve global problems. So look for the type of generalizations made by the author. If they go too far beyond the research, the author is too egocentric. Or the conclusions might be too narrow, too specific to the research. You are, after all, looking for some creativity from the researcher.

Defective conclusions are either too broad, too specific, or non-existent. Substandard conclusions, leave you hanging—you have no sense of completeness. The adequate conclusion has a sense of finality and closure, and derives directly from the problem.

You now know this article backwards and forwards. You have a feeling about the article—good, bad, or indifferent—a feeling generated by the end of the report. Now let's see how objective that feeling really is.

Go back to the very beginning of the report. Get out a pencil and paper. Start at the top left-hand side of the paper and list each of the major portions of the research report: *problem, sample, methods, analysis, findings/conclusions.* Across the top of the paper list your headings: *defective, substandard* and *adequate.* Now check off under which heading each section of the article falls. Add up the number of checks you have made in the defective column and multiply by one. Add the checks in the substandard column and multiply by two. Multiply the sum in the adequate column by three. Total the scores. If you gave the report at least 12 points, it is adequate. If the report scored from 8 to 11, it is substandard. If the score fell below 8 you have a defective study.

Check your score against the feeling you had after you had thoroughly analyzed the article. Do they agree, or is the score totally discrepant from your feeling? If similar, you have just verified the reliability of your feelings. But since feelings and impressions are not always reliable indicators of how good each aspect of the report was, use your objective scoring method until your feelings and the scores agree consistently.

WHERE DOES THE CRITIQUE BELONG?

It may surprise you to find out, after all of this work, that the critique doesn't *belong* anywhere. Your critique is for *you* as part of your development as an authority in this area of research. You won't find critiques at the end of research proposals as appendixes. You won't include your critique as a part of your proposal. But you will use the results of your critiques throughout your research plan, data collection, analysis of data, and final written report. As specific entities, they don't *belong* anywhere. As a process critical to your development as a researcher, they belong everywhere and all the time.

Just as you have learned about the research proposal, there is a difference between the process of getting somewhere and the final end point or result of that process. Your critiques are a part of the process of building your proposal. Thus, you will cite either in your bibliography or list of references, every *adequate* piece of research you have actually used to develop your proposal. You will reference inadequate or substandard reports only when that is all that was available, specifying in what way they were inadequate and your reason for using them anyway. In order to do all of this with reasonable veracity, you must have *critiqued* what you read.

No one can, or will, do this for you; it is your responsibility. But the results are worth it.

RECOMMENDED READING

Fleming, Juanita W., and Hayter, Jean. "Reading Research Reports Critically." *Nursing Outlook* 22 (1974): 172–176.

Fox, David. *Fundamentals of Research in Nursing,* Chapter 13. Appleton-Century-Crofts, 1970.

Leininger, Madeleine M. "The Research Critique: Nature, Function and Art." *Communicating Nursing Research: The Research Critique,* pp. 21–23. Boulder, Colorado: Western Interstate Commission for Higher Education, July, 1968.

Notter, Lucille. *Essentials of Nursing Research,* Chapter 10. New York: Springer Publishing Co., 1974.

Stetler, Cheryl B., and Marram, Gwen. "Evaluating Research Findings for Applicability in Practice." *Nursing Outlook* 24 (Sept. 1976): 559–563.

NLN Research and Studies Service. "Search or Research: Criteria for a Research Report." *Nursing Outlook* 12 (August 1964): 60.

VI.

The Purpose of the Study: Answering the Question

LEVEL I: The Purpose Written as a Declarative Statement

LEVEL II: The Purpose Written as a Question

LEVEL III: The Purpose Written as a Hypothesis

Rewriting the Question as the Purpose

Why state the purpose of the study when the question has already been well developed and supported by a logical argument? Of what use is a statement of purpose?

The main benefit of *the purpose* is that it says *exactly* what you intend to do to answer your question. It should include one of two things: 1) what you will do to *collect data* (for example, observe and describe, listen and describe) or 2) what you will *observe or measure* (for example, age, occupation, self-image). Then you must include some information about *where* the data will be collected (the setting of the study), and *who* the subjects will be. These *three* aspects of the purpose are stated in such a way that the research design follows logically.

There are three ways to state the purpose of a study: 1) as a declarative statement; 2) as a question; and 3) as a hypothesis. The appropriate method to choose depends on the kind of question you asked and the extent of your knowledge about the problem. These two factors are closely related, as you know. You asked a Level I (what, where, when, who) question when you were able to find very little information about your topic. You asked a more complex Level II question (What is the difference . . .) when you were able to find literature describing your concepts and providing some theoretical background for your study. You asked a Level III (why or if-then) question when you were able to develop a sound conceptual framework for your study and find research on which to build your idea. Let's look at the relationship between the purpose and the complexity of the question.

LEVEL I: THE PURPOSE WRITTEN AS A DECLARATIVE STATEMENT

When your knowledge about the research problem is limited because little or no prior research was done, your study will focus on the search for information. Your question is a *who, what, when* or *where* question at the simplest level. In this case, your purpose *must be* a declarative statement, giving direction for *what* is to be done, *where*, and *with whom*. Look at the following questions:

1. *What* do patients like and dislike about nurses?
2. *When* do dying patients begin to withdraw from their families?
3. *Who* are the patients that nurses classify as "crocks"?

Let's assume that little or nothing is known about the topics of these questions. There is no theory, no previous research upon which to base a study, therefore the basic purpose will be to *explore*. Instead of starting with concepts and a conceptual framework, you will develop concepts as your end product. Now, how does the statement of purpose differ from the original question?

The purpose must state exactly *what* you intend to do, *where* you intend to do it, and with *whom,* in order to answer the question. Purposes that are declarative statements *always* result in description. Take the first question above, "*What* do patients like and dislike about nurses?" The purpose becomes:

> The purpose of this study is to describe and classify the likes and dislikes expressed by patients about the nurses on all three shifts of the orthopedic unit.

In developing the problem from this question, no information was found relating to the kinds of likes and dislikes. This study will explore what they are. The results (or answer) will be description and classification. A conceptual framework that ties together the resultant ideas about patients' likes and dislikes will be the outcome of the study.

In the second example, "*When* do dying patients begin to withdraw from their families?", a similar situation exists. There is no previous research, or perhaps all the literature deals with the family's withdrawal from the patient rather than the patient's behavior. The purpose of this study might look like this:

> The purpose of this study is to observe and describe the stage of the dying process where the terminal oncology patient begins to withdraw from his family.

In exploring one aspect of dying, this study will result in description and possibly some predictions about contributory factors that might be tested in further studies. However, at present there is insufficient information to consider a withdrawal stage as a concept about the dying process. No predictions are possible about findings; therefore the purpose can only be stated as a declarative statement as to *what* will be done, *where,* and *with whom.*

"*Who* are the patients that nurses classify as 'crocks'?" This question obviously comes from a real situation in which the researcher observed nurses classifying patients into categories according to some "unwritten" criteria. No theories exist that explain this phenomenon, and no description can be found listing the characteristics of the patients involved. The appropriate level for this study, therefore, is to explore and describe, and the purpose would be the following:

> The purpose of this study is to describe the characteristics of patients whom nurses on a medical-surgical unit have classified as "crock."

The purpose explains what the researcher will do. The setting and the sample are described in general terms (specifics are given later in the proposal). The results of this study might very well develop the idea of "crock" into a conceptual framework within which to study nurse-patient interaction.

LEVEL II: THE PURPOSE WRITTEN AS A QUESTION

When you know enough about your topic to know what you will be observing, but not enough to make a prediction about your findings, your purpose should be stated as a question. How much knowledge is enough but not too much? How can you tell if your study should be at this level?

Let's look at some sample questions:

1. What is the relationship between age and rate of learning in auto-tutorial settings?
2. What is the difference between the role perceptions of patients who were emergency admissions and those who were scheduled for admission?

These are both *what* questions, but at a different level than the exploratory kind. These questions start with concepts about which the researcher obviously has some knowledge, because the question asks about relationships between concepts or among ideas within a concept. The immediate difference between these questions and the previous exploratory kind is that these begin with a concept.

The concepts from which the first question emerges are maturation and learning. These concepts had to have been discussed during the development of the problem to clarify the researcher's frame of reference. You know that the researcher's concept of maturation was based on Eriksen's stages of development, and that the concept of learning stemmed from stimulus-response theory. However, nothing in the literature gave any basis for predicting the effect of maturation on learning; therefore, the question asked, "What is the relationship?"

This question raises another point: the use of the age variable to represent the concept of maturation. A variable is anything that varies, or any property that takes on different values. In other words, it is something that can be measured. Because a concept cannot be directly measured, it must first be defined in measurable terms as a variable (or series of variables) that will, when measured, represent the concept as it has been described. (See Chapter VII.) In this case, maturation has been described in such a way that the age of the individual will represent his or her level of maturation. Other aspects of maturation that might be measured by psychological or physiological variables are not being considered in this study.

One of the side effects of the statement of purpose is that it limits the study to that which the purpose specifies. This prevents the researcher from being sidetracked once the study has begun. Therefore, any statement of purpose should be as specific as possible to make the rest of the proposal easier to develop.

The purpose of the study from the first question can be stated as follows: The purpose of this study is to answer the question, is there a relationship between age and rate of learning pharmacology among nurses in an auto-tutorial program? The difference between this purpose, written as a question, and the initial research question is that *this is a yes/no question.* The answer will be *yes* or *no* and will be determined by the data. The *significance* of the answer will also be determined, so that the answer to this level of question always requires some statistical analysis.

This level of purpose also leads to a descriptive design, but is not exploring "unknown territory" as was the case with the declarative statement of purpose.

Let's look at another example of stating the purpose as a question.

"What is the difference between the role perceptions of patients who were emergency admissions and those who were scheduled admissions?"

The conceptual framework behind this question is that of role, and more specifically, that of role-taking. The question is looking for relationships among ideas within the concept of role-taking, the ideas of preparation and nonpreparation as they influence the patient's role perception. Because of the level of knowledge in this area, it is possible once again to specify exactly which concepts and variables will be observed. It is not possible to predict how they will influence one another, or what the outcome will be. So stating the purpose as a question is appropriate. It would look like this:

The purpose of this study is to answer the question, Is there a difference in the role perceptions of patients who have undergone elective abdominal surgery versus those who have had emergency abdominal surgery on the third postoperative day?

The result of this study would reflect the significance of the *yes* or *no* answer obtained from the data. Since this question is looking for the difference between groups of patients, you are safe in assuming that role perceptions of patients have already been described in previous studies. If they had not, then it would not be appropriate to start at this level.

LEVEL III: THE PURPOSE WRITTEN AS A HYPOTHESIS

When you have enough information to predict the outcome of your study and your intent is to test the significance of your prediction, your question is at Level III and the purpose of your study will be stated as a hypothesis.

A hypothesis is simply a statement that asserts a relationship between two or more variables. Hypotheses are only possible in studies that are based on conceptual or theoretical frameworks; they must be supported by the argument developed during the definition of the problem. Although hypotheses are sometimes referred to as "hunches" or "guesses," they are never just pulled out of thin air; rather, they are *calculated* guesses that can be supported by theory and previous research.

Sometimes hypotheses specify causal relationships, but more often they simply specify a relationship between two or more variables. The hypothesis will state either that these variables will be found to exist together, or that a change in one will be associated with a change in another. The reason behind the hypothesis must always be explained in the rationale for the study, and must be based on a sound conceptual or theoretical base. In the case of a cause-and-effect relationship, the base *must* be theory.

Take the following research questions:

1. *If* pregnant women are given antibiotics during the first trimester, *then* what is the effect on the development of the bone structure of the fetus?
2. *Why* is authoritarianism more prevalent among long-term psychiatric nurses than among medical-surgical nurses?
3. *Why* is an increase in significant life changes associated with a higher incidence of heart disease in middle-aged women?

The first of these research questions combines theory of growth during fetal development with biochemical theory, specifically recent studies of the calcium-binding effect of some antibiotics, and proposes a cause-and-effect relationship. The purpose of the study would be stated as follows:

The purpose of this study is to test the following hypothesis: The incidence of bone structure deformities will be significantly higher among the newborn infants of subjects who were treated with Calciomycetin than those who received no Calciomycetin during the first trimester of pregnancy.

This hypothesis predicts a causal relationship between Calciomycetin and bone deformities in newborn infants. This prediction can be supported by theory and previous research and needs to be tested through research in order to become an established relationship. Few nursing studies deal with cause-and-effect relationships, because we deal with people in social and cultural settings in which multiple variables are interacting. It becomes very difficult to isolate the effect of one variable in order to prove its causal effect on another variable. Thus, nursing hypotheses usually predict relationships and not causes.

The second question is an example: *Why* is authoritarianism more prevalent among long-term psychiatric nurses than among medical-surgical nurses?

Because it asks *why*, this question implies that measures of authoritarianism among psychiatric nurses are higher than those for medical-surgical nurses. This statement must be supported not only by a conceptual framework for authoritarianism, but also by previous research that describes authoritarianism in these nurses. Theoretically, a case can be built to explain why. Now, by controlling as many factors as possible that might interfere, it is necessary to test the relationship. The purpose would be:

> The purpose of this study is to test the following hypothesis: Long-term psychiatric nurses in an inpatient setting will have significantly higher scores for authoritarianism than medical-surgical nurses who have been on the job for the same length of time.

This hypothesis predicts that a high degree of authoritarianism will be found in psychiatric nursing. It does *not* say that a propensity for authoritarianism *causes* nurses to become psychiatric nurses, nor does it propose that being a psychiatric nurse causes a high degree of authoritarianism. But it does propose that the two are related and will be found to exist together. The conceptual framework will explain why.

The third question proposes a relationship between significant life changes and the incidence of heart disease in middle-aged women. It also implies that an increase in one is associated with an increase in the other. The purpose states:

> The purpose of this study is to test the following hypothesis: An increase in significant life changes in middle-aged women will be associated with a higher incidence of heart disease.

Although it may be inferred from this purpose that life changes are contributing to a higher incidence of heart disease, no direct cause-and-effect relationship is stated. Because of the complexity of interacting factors, no one factor such as life changes could be isolated to test for a causal relationship. However, continued associative relationships will lend support to the theory.

In all of these studies designed to test hypotheses, the proposal must include the plan for the statistical analysis that will either support or refute your hypothesis. (See chapter XIII.)

REWRITING THE QUESTION AS THE PURPOSE

Now you are ready to look at your research question—your definition of the problem—and decide on the purpose of your study. You know whether you are starting from a conceptual framework or whether you hope to end with one. You know whether you are tilling virgin soil or whether you are building on developed land. You know if you are searching for or predicting the outcome. By process of elimination, you are ready to state your purpose.

VII.

Defining Your Terms

In the discussion of writing a research question, the question was divided into its component parts: the stem question and the topic. The stem question directs the research process, while the topic is the actual focus of the study. The same stem and topic are then used to formulate the purpose of the study. The literature review has been in relation to the topic—who has studied it, what was said about it, how the variables were measured, and whether or not the variables you are using have been put together in the same way before. The information you found on the topic has helped you to determine the exact purpose of your study. Now you need to be more precise about the variables themselves.

Recall that in chapter VI we defined a variable as anything that varies, or any property that takes on different values. Before you can define your variables, you must decide exactly what you want to know. Suppose you are interested in anxiety. You know that anxiety can be short-term or long-term, acute or chronic, normal or abnormal, perceived by an observer or reported by an individual, manifest or latent, mild or severe. The aspect of anxiety in which you are interested and the ways in which it varies is what you are going to measure. Your statement about this becomes your *definition of terms*. The aspect of anxiety that you are going to measure and the method you will use constitutes its *operational definition*. Operational definitions describe *what* you are going to measure and *how* you will measure it. They involve deleting all aspects of the variable except those in which you are interested, and then specifying how it will be measured.

As an example, your definition of anxiety might read: "vague feelings of alarm that persons report when faced with a stressful situation," or it could read: "behavioral manifestations of persons subjected to stress, which can be identified by facial grimaces, muscle tensing and palmar sweating." Still another definition might say, "a trait possessed by all persons to some degree, which is reflected in their responses to questions about their view of life in general."

Each of these definitions measures a completely different concept of anxiety. The first one measures a person's report of how they feel. The second measures an observer's perception of the individual's behavior. The third requires that the researcher infer how the individual feels from his or her responses to questions. None of these is a perfect measure; none is better than the others.

Your operational definition must specify what *you* want to study and how *you* want to study it, and nothing more.

During the development of the problem, you dealt with the whole realm of literature and theory about anxiety. You decided which frame of reference you wanted to assume. Now you must eliminate everything except that which fits your frame of reference and represents what you will be measuring. In other words, the operational definition isolates the central component of the variable under study and *deletes* all other components of that variable.

Theoretically, your operational definitions can be anything you want them to be, but you should use some evaluative criteria when developing them. They should have logical, empirical meaning and should define your concepts explicitly and precisely. In addition, they should relate directly to the theory upon which they are based.

EXAMPLE: Stress is defined as the number and severity of surgical procedures an individual has undergone during the past five years.

Strictly speaking, you are free to define stress in this way for your study. However, you must recognize that this definition is not generally used for stress, and in fact, has no relation to any theory of stress. Therefore, you need to ask yourself, What do I really want to know? If you want to measure stress according to a conceptual framework that you have developed from some of the literature you have read, you need to rethink your definition. However, if what you really want to know is the patient's previous experience with surgical trauma, keep your definition but call it something else.

TYPES OF VARIABLES

When the research plan hypothesizes relationships between variables, it is necessary to clarify the expected relationships by categorizing the variables as *independent* or *dependent*. The terms come from experimental research, where an independent or experimental variable is introduced into a controlled setting, and the result is measured. This result —the response to the independent variable—is called the *dependent* variable. Changes in the dependent variable are considered to be "caused by" the introduction of the independent variable. When the hypothesis does not predict a causal relationship, but simply an associative one, as is often the case in Level II descriptive surveys, the independent variable can still be identified as the one that came first in time and is thought to be affecting the response (dependent variable). For instance, in the hypothesis, "Turnover of staff nurses is significantly higher on units where the leadership style is authoritarian," a relationship is predicted between turnover of staff and authoritarian leadership. No cause-and-effect relationship is specified, because there are too many other possible variables that could be working with authoritarianism to bring about turnover. However, it is implied that authoritarianism is affecting turnover. Therefore, authoritarianism is the independent variable and turnover is the dependent variable. To test this hypothesis, it would be necessary to find at least two groups of nursing leaders, those who are authoritarian and those who are not, and then look at the difference in turnover of their nursing staffs.

One easy way of differentiating between independent and dependent variables is to remember that *independent* means to stand alone, and *dependent* means to rely on, or depend on, the independent variable.

Extraneous variables are all those which are not of direct interest to you as the researcher, but which could be creating an effect on the variables that you are measuring. In studies where hypotheses are tested, the major purpose of the research design is to control the effect of extraneous variables so that the effect of the independent variable on the dependent variable can be estimated. If you were trying to test the effect of authoritarian leadership on nursing staff turnover, many extraneous variables would need to be controlled. Some of these might be the nurses' age, educational background, marital status, and number of children. Any or all of these variables could affect the turnover of the nursing staff and therefore must be controlled by the design.

DEFINING THE INDEPENDENT VARIABLE

In research, the independent variable is the characteristic by which the subgroups in the sample are distinguished. In other words, the researcher must be able to divide the sample into alternative groups based on this variable. For example, authoritarian/nonauthoritarian and smoking/nonsmoking are both instances where the independent variable is divided into two categories. Or you might wish to establish more than two categories: light, medium, and heavy smokers, based on the number of cigarettes smoked per day. In some studies, the independent variable might be divided into numerous precise classes, such as multiple dosage levels of a drug or exact monthly income. In defining the independent variable, the researcher decides on the categories for the sample. In doing this, there are three important objectives to keep in mind.

First, the various subdivisions or categories of the variable must be easily distinguished from one another, and they must be mutually exclusive. There may not be a case where a subject would easily fit into more than one category at a time. The number of cigarettes per day constituting a medium smoker must be clearly distinguishable from that constituting a light smoker. The method of measurement for the categories must be clearly defined so that others reading the study can replicate them. If the number of cigarettes are to be counted for a week and then divided by seven days, it must be clearly stated and understood.

Second, the distinction between the categories should mean something in terms of the research problem. If age categories are developed to test the idea that children of different ages respond differently to health teaching, then the age categories must have some meaning in light of developmental theory. It is not enough just to set age categories by five-year increments; the categories selected must relate to the theory behind the study.

Third, the definition of the independent variable must remain constant during the data collection as well as during the analysis of the data. If a nursing intervention is introduced to reduce pain in postoperative patients, and partway through the study it becomes apparent that the intervention is not working, it may not be increased or decreased, nor may it be changed to another intervention, in order to change the results. A study that shows *no* difference between the intervention and nonintervention groups makes an important contribution to nursing theory.

A more subtle alteration in the definition of the independent variable can occur in this example. If several members of the nursing staff are required to carry out the intervention, perhaps even the entire staff of a particular unit, it may happen that some nurses do not follow the protocol of the study unless the researcher is actually present. When this happens, an alternate version of the independent variable is present and its effect is being combined with that of the true variable. If the researcher is unaware of the problem, the relationship that emerges between the independent and dependent variables might be a spurious one.

The definition of the independent variable is critical to studies in which the purpose is stated as a question or a hypothesis. When a study is testing the independent variable as the cause or the dependent variable as the effect of the independent variable, then the description and definition of the independent variable is mandatory. On the other hand, in descriptive studies all variables are assumed to be independent. This is simply due to the lack of knowledge about the variables. Therefore, when a variable's status is unknown, it must be treated *as if* it were independent.

MEASUREMENT OF VARIABLES

Variables can be grouped at certain levels of precision according to your operational definitions and your measurement of the responses. There are four levels of precision: *nominal, ordinal, interval,* and *ratio.*

1. *Nominal Scale.* When objects or events are classified into two or more categories, and no difference in magnitude or value exists between categories, they are being studied on a nominal scale. The only

specified relationship between the categories is that they are different from one another. There is no suggestion of quantity. Nominal scales are appropriate to classifications, typologies, and yes/no responses. The type of variables that fit this scale are things like occupation, race, marital status, religion, type of illness, cause of death. Nominal scales vary in size from those having just two categories, such as sex, to those with numerous categories, such as a typology of medical diagnoses. The data collected with nominal scales are called frequency data. The number or percentage of persons falling into each category are tabulated. Contrasts and comparisons of the categories can then be made. For example, you could look at marital status, occupation, and cause of death, and perhaps find a trend among single, unemployed suicides. Your independent variable will frequently be on a nominal scale. Smokers/nonsmokers and authoritarian/nonauthoritarian are two examples. However, when you decide to develop *degrees* of authoritarianism, you no longer have nominal data.

2. *Ordinal Scales.* Just as the nominal scale refers to *naming* data, the ordinal scale refers to *ordering* data. Here, differences in magnitude are assigned to each category. Instead of having two categories of authoritarian and nonauthoritarian, you now have a scale starting at *none* and proceeding to *little, moderate,* and *extensive.* Note that positions on the scale are in order. There can be any number of positions on an ordinal scale, but the actual distances from one point to the next are not *measureable.*

EXAMPLE: Strongly agree/agree/neutral/disagree/strongly disagree.

This five-point scale is often used to measure attitudes. Subjects are asked to choose the point on the scale that comes closest to reflecting their attitudes towards a statement. The scale is ordered according to the degree of the subjects' agreement with the statement. However, no inferences can be drawn about the actual difference in the attitude of a subject who checks *agree* versus one who checks *strongly agree* or *disagree.* Nevertheless, many statistical tests can be performed with ordinal data, which are ranked.

3. *Interval Scales.* These differ from ordinal scales in that on these scales there are numerically equal distances between the points. The intervals can be added and subtracted and will provide accurate information about the difference between the subjects' positions.

You can determine how much more one category is than another on an interval scale. To make such comparisons, you need a unit of measurement and an arbitrary zero point. For example, a subject's temperature in degrees Fahrenheit is an interval scale where $0°$ F is the origin and $1°$ is the unit of measurement.

4. *Ratio Scales.* The highest level of measurement is ratio measurement. It differs from the interval scale only in that a ratio scale has

an *absolute* zero with empirical meaning. A zero measurement on a scale indicates that none of the property being measured exists at that point. All arithmetic operations are possible with this scale, including multiplication and division. Numbers on the scale indicate the actual amounts of the variable being measured. Examples of ratio scales are weight, height, and time.

Most nursing research utilizes nominal and ordinal scales. These are the most commonly-used scales in behavioral and social research. Increasing use is also being made of interval and ratio level data, especially in nursing research influenced by the biological and physical sciences. In a later chapter, you will see how the measurement scale of your variables affects the possibilities for data analysis.

TERMS THAT NEED DEFINITION

When you write the purpose of your study, you are stating exactly what it is you intend to study about your chosen topic. Because of the specific nature of the purpose, every important word—nouns, verbs, adverbs, and adjectives—that it contains should be operationally defined. If you use words in your definitions that need to be defined also, then add those to the list. The economy of words in a purpose necessitates *operational definitions*.

This chapter has focused on the operational definition of the independent and dependent variables as the critical issue for the project. Remember, in a descriptive study, *all* variables are assumed to be independent. Therefore, all terms need definition. In an experimental design, you as investigator are in total and complete control (at least, theoretically) over the independent variable; therefore, you must know everything you can about it. Your study describes the resulting effect on the dependent variable. Thus, the independent and dependent variables are the crux of the proposal and the central terms that need definition. You also need to define the possible extraneous variables to show your reader that you have taken them into account.

RECOMMENDED READING

Johnson, B. A., Johnson, J. E., and Dumas, R. G. "Research in Nursing Practice: The Problem of Uncontrolled Situational Variables." *Nursing Research* 19 (July–August 1970): 337–342.

Kerlinger, Fred N. *Foundations of Behavioral Research.* New York: Holt, Rinehart and Winston, 1964.

VIII.

The Research Design: Blueprint for Action

Designing Your Study from the Question

Descriptive Designs
1. Exploratory Descriptive Designs
2. Descriptive Survey Designs

Explanatory Designs
1. Explanatory Survey Designs
2. Experimental Designs

The preceding chapters have taken you through the process of deciding *what* you want to study. The remaining chapters will help you to decide *how* to study it. You are ready to take the work you have already done—your stem question, your topic, your operational definitions, and your statement of purpose—and lay them out into a working plan, a blueprint for action.

Now is the time to start thinking about the details. What should you call your design? Is it an experiment or is it a survey? What will your sample be like? Where will you find subjects? What will they be like? How many will you need? Where will you find tools to measure your variables? All these, and many more, are questions you must answer in your blueprint.

As with any blueprint, you start with an overall picture of the design, and then go on to show close-up pictures of each section. In that way, you don't get bogged down in detail before you have visualized the end result. If you tried to design a kitchen by starting with a detailed plan for the spice cupboard and then tried to fit the rest of the kitchen around it, you would be in trouble. Similarly, the research plan will suffer if you start by minutely describing the sample before you know what the overall plan is to be. The result would be a research design planned to fit the sample instead of a sample that meets the needs of the design.

Let's start by discussing the overall design.

DESIGNING YOUR STUDY FROM THE QUESTION

All research designs fall into one of two categories: descriptive or explanatory. Descriptive designs result in a description of the data, whether in words, pictures, charts, or tables, and whether the data analysis shows statistical relationships or is merely descriptive. Explanatory designs result in inferences being drawn from the data that explain the relationships between the variables.

What, when, where, and *who* questions invariably lead to descriptive designs; *why* and *if-then* questions are *always* explanatory. In addition, if your purpose fits the declarative statement category, you have an exploratory descriptive study, whereas the purpose written as a question leads to a descriptive survey design. On the other hand, the purpose as a hypothesis leads only to an explanatory design. Thus, the choice of which type of design to use was made when you finalized your question, and was carved in cement when you stated the purpose of your study. Therefore, all you need to do now is give it a name.

Why do you need a label? What is the purpose of a design?

The design is a set of instructions to the researcher to gather and analyze data in certain ways, so that there will be control over *who* and *what* are to be studied. Unwanted or extraneous variables can be controlled; the variance of the specified variables is enhanced; and the possibility of error in measurement is minimized. In other words, the design helps you to isolate the variables you are interested in from all other variables, and to measure them accurately so that your data are reliable and valid.

Once again, all designs fall into two major categories; descriptive or explanatory. The choice of which kind to do is made during the development of the problem. When you read about your topic and found out what is known about it, the choice of design for your question was made. If your question turned out to be at level 1 or 2, the design will be descriptive; if you have a level 3 question, it will take an explanatory design to answer it.

The design chosen must be the *best* way to answer the question. *Best* in this case means the one that fits with the level of the question. Variables about which nothing is known must be questioned at a very basic level, and the answer must provide *description* of those variables. When there is considerable knowledge about the action of the variables, both independently and in association with others, the question will ask for an *explanation* of the action, and the design will test the explanation.

The design always goes forward from what has gone before. The only exception to this rule occurs in replication studies. If you question the results of previous research, and feel that they require further support, your study may replicate the previous research. In this case, you must follow the design *exactly* as it was in the original study, rather than build on the results of the original study.

DESCRIPTIVE DESIGNS

No matter what method is chosen to collect the data, all descriptive designs have one thing in common: they must provide descriptions of the variables in order to answer the question. The type of description that results from the design does, however, depend on how much information the researcher had about the topic prior to data collection.

Rather than creating numerous levels of descriptive designs, it makes more sense to look at the design in the same way that we looked at the question. Level I questions with little or no prior knowledge of the topic lead to exploratory descriptive designs. Level II questions, where the variables are known but their action cannot be predicted, lead to descriptive survey designs.

Exploratory Descriptive Designs

When the purpose of a study is exploration, a flexible research design is needed, one that provides an opportunity to examine all aspects of the problem. As the variables become apparent, the researcher may have to change direction. Ideas occur as data are collected and examined. The key to a good exploratory design is *flexibility*.

We emphasize throughout the book that the research process is dependent on what is known about the topic. The word *exploratory* indicates that not much is known, which means that a survey of the literature failed to reveal any significant research in the area. Thus you cannot build upon the work of others; you *must* explore the topic for yourself.

Even though we talk about the exploratory study as an entity in itself, it should be remembered that it is an initial step in the development of new knowledge. Because of the flexibility of this type of design, very few, if any, variables are under the researcher's control. They are said to be under the control of the *situation;* in other words, observed as they happen, or as the researcher comes upon them. As a result, no inferences can be drawn from the data. The data may lead to suggestions of hypotheses for further study, or an idea for a conceptual framework to explain the action of the variables, but the exploratory question *must* be followed by higher level questions if new knowledge is to be gained.

In nursing research, there are many topics for which the level of knowledge is such that exploratory studies are required. For instance, a research question might be, "*What* is the reaction of patients to being transferred from room to room during hospitalization?" This question looks like an exploratory question. If the literature review reveals no information on this topic, the purpose of your study will be to explore and describe patients' reactions to being moved from room to room during a hospital stay. In this type of study, you may *not* ask, "What is the *effect* of moving patients from room to room?" In order to ask questions about effect, you must know the cause and have sufficient information to predict the effect; or you may know the effect, in which case you must be able to predict the cause. Either option requires a lot of information. You do not have this type of information in our present example. You have no idea whether moving patients has any effect on anything at all. And if there is an effect, you have no idea of its extent. Perhaps it will be temporary annoyance; a mild disorientation; a severe setback in convalescence, an increase in sensory disturbances; or a loss of social relationships—the list of possibilities could fill volumes. In order to find out what the patient's reaction actually is, you will have to explore all these possibilities. That means asking open-ended questions and being prepared to shift gears depending on the patient's initial responses. You will need to observe patients being moved and describe what you see; you will need to interview patients and families and ask what their reactions are; you will want to question nurses, ward clerks, physicians, and others who are in contact with the patient to see what their experiences have been. Your methods and questions will change depending on what you find out as you go along. Thus it is imperative that the design be *flexible.*

The results of this study will provide detailed descriptions of all the observations made by the researcher, arranged in some kind of order. Conclusions drawn from the data would include some educated guesses or hypotheses for further study. A relationship between the observations made and a concept such as territorialism might be proposed. Or perhaps a relationship to systems theory might be seen. Further research would be required to test these proposals. This is the purpose of exploratory research.

Descriptive Survey Designs

Questions at level 2 ask, "What is the relationship between or among variables?" You know what the variables are, and you know how to measure them, so you are beyond the scope of an exploratory study. The variables you are interested in have been studied before, either independently, as in an exploratory study, or with other variables, so that there is sufficient information to ask a question about the relationship between them. You are able to relate the variables in your study to a concept or conceptual framework, so that the study does build on previous work. The major consideration is *accuracy* in the measurement of the variables.

Designs for studies at level 2 require a descriptive survey. The question asks about the relationship between or among variables; the design must dictate how the variables are to be measured in testing the relationship. In this type of design the variables are partly controlled by the situation, as they were in exploratory designs, but they are also partly controlled by the investigator, who chooses a sample for the study. The other variables are taken as they come; the investigator has no control over them. For example, in a study of the relationship between educational level of nurses and the ability to make sound judgments about patient care, the investigator controls the first variable by selecting a sample of nurses with all types of educational background. The judgments of these nurses are then examined in relation to their soundness. This latter variable will be controlled by the situation, not the investigator. The nurses' judgments will be examined and evaluated as they occur; the purpose of the study will be accomplished by seeing if the occurrence of sound judgment is related to educational background.

Do not fall into the trap of thinking that a survey must be something similar to the Gallup poll of political views, which surveys a random sample of the nations' voters. The poll is a type of survey, but surveys cover all types of studies where a group of people are examined to see how they compare on two or more variables. There are many types of descriptive surveys. Some look at one population, such as nurses, to see what their attitude is toward some issue, such as abortion or women's rights. Others take two or more groups, such as blacks, whites, and Chicanos, and see if they differ on some variable, such as life expectancy or the incidence of a particular health problem. Still others take a small patient population, such as renal dialysis patients, and study their coping mechanisms in relation to their acceptance or rejection of a transplanted kidney. All of these are descriptive surveys. The answer is in descriptive form, just as with exploratory designs, but this time the description is of the relationship between the variables rather than of the variables themselves.

EXPLANATORY DESIGNS

The common element in all explanatory designs is that they attempt to establish causal relationships. Explanatory studies come from third-level questions, which started by asking *why* or *if-then*. The variables must have been studied sufficiently so that their interaction can be predicted and explained by a conceptual or theoretical framework. These studies are designed to test hypotheses; therefore, the major consideration must be the control of the variables so that their influence on one another can be determined. The end product of an explanatory study is *explanation;* this explanation is directed at the development of causal relationships.

Terms like *cause-and-effect* are frequently used in the popular sense, rather than the research sense. There is nothing mysterious about a cause. It is not a supernatural force that makes things happen, nor is it likely to be a single factor that will create an effect by itself. Rather, a cause-and-effect idea identifies a sequence of events that provides a sensible explanation of how and why things happen the way they do. In order to support this idea, criteria have been developed for testing hypotheses so that the causal sequence can be inferred. These criteria include: (1) presence of a co-variation between the cause and the effect, (2) the cause having preceded the effect in time and (3) elimination of other possible explanations for the relationship between the cause and effect. If these three criteria can be met, then a causal relationship has been established.

What is meant by a causal relationship? A casual relationship identifies one characteristic or event that with other factors determines another characteristic or event. *Explanatory designs* provide the strategy for examining the evidence to support (or refute) the hypothesis of the causal relationship.

The two major categories of explanatory designs are *explanatory surveys* and *experimental designs.* These differ in the type of control the researcher has over the variables and whether the focus of attention is of the cause or the effect.

In explanatory surveys, the researcher controls the variables by selecting a sample in which they exist. As the researcher, you start with the effect, or dependent variable, and set about to find the cause, or independent variable. In experimental designs, on the other hand, all the variables are under the researcher's strict control. Here, you start with the causal variable and manipulate it to see if you can create the effect. Both are attempting to support the causal relationship by looking at the three criteria for causality, but the approach in each case is quite different.

Explanatory Survey Designs

Many research questions ask about variables that cannot be subjected to experimental manipulation, either because the variables cannot be manipulated or because to look at them outside of their natural setting would be meaningless. For example, to look at factors leading to mental illness, it would be impossible to isolate a single factor such as poverty and manipulate it to see if it results in mental illness. An experimental design would require that subjects be assigned to groups placed in different levels of poverty. After the specified length of time had passed, the groups would be examined to see if mental illness had developed. The absurdity of such an approach is obvious.

Rather than using experimentation to develop a causal sequence leading to mental illness, you would start with the effect, mental illness. Selecting a sample possessing this variable would be the first step. Then you would look for variables that might lead to mental illness. You might find a significant relationship between poverty and mental illness. You might also establish that poverty precedes mental illness in time. You have now met two of the three criteria for establishing a causal relationship, and have only to rule out alternative explanations for the apparent relationship. Here you might run into some difficulty. You might discover that well-to-do persons are less likely to be diagnosed as mentally ill even with the same symptoms as the persons at the bottom of the poverty scale. The type of health care available to persons of different economic levels is different, as is educational opportunity and many other factors. However, this is the chance you take when trying to establish causality. Alternative explanations are always strong possibilities in explanatory surveys, since subjects differ on many factors, only a few of which can be controlled. There is no way to equate groups without random assignment, and, of course, no way to do random assignment in a survey design.

Although proof of causality beyond a shadow of a doubt cannot be established in an explanatory survey, it is possible to accumulate extensive evidence to support causality. Much of the research on cigarette smoking and lung cancer was done through the use of explanatory surveys. No experimental research has or, hopefully, ever will be done with human subjects to see if lung cancer can be created by introducing cigarette smoking. But by showing that cigarette smoking is the one variable that stands out as preponderant in persons with lung cancer, support grows for the theory that the disease can be caused by smoking.

There are many variables of interest to nursing researchers that cannot be experimentally manipulated. Often the concepts that are conceived of as being causal are things like attitudes or beliefs or behaviors—all factors of interest in relation to health, illness, response to treatment, and other effects that nurses are interested in studying. The explanatory survey can be of great value in the study of these variables.

Experimental Designs

What is an experiment? It is a study in which the researcher has control over the independent variable and over the assignment of subjects to different experimental conditions. True experiments are conducted in controlled laboratories where the effects of an independent variable are examined, in isolation from other factors. Experiments also can be carried out in natural settings if the researcher has enough control over the environment.

Some of the problems that arise in explanatory surveys in establishing causal relationships can be eliminated in experimental designs. Problems such as the possibility that the cause and effect are in fact reversed and the dependent variable is actually creating the independent variable, are difficult to rule out in a survey design. For instance, it may be found that nurses who have close contact with sex-change surgery patients have more positive attitudes toward these patients than do nurses who have little or no contact with such patients. This appears to support the theory that frequent contact creates favorable attitudes. However, there is really no way to rule out the possibility that the favorable attitude *preceded* the close contact, and that in fact the causal sequence is reversed. Nurses who already have favorable attitudes towards transsexuals and sex-change surgery may be more likely to choose to work with those patients.

In an experimental design, there is no question about what created the effect, or which came first. The first and foremost criterion for an experimental design is that the independent variable is introduced to the sample by the researcher. The rest of the design simply sets up rules by which other variables can be kept from interfering.

One of the best ways that an experimental design can rule out the interference of other variables is through the use of control groups. By assigning subjects randomly to either an experimental or a control group, it is possible to have two equivalent groups at the beginning of the experiment. By administering the experimental variable to one of these groups, it is possible to attribute any change that occurs in the experimental group and not in the control group to the effect of this variable.

The number of experimental and control groups to be used in one design can vary widely and will depend very much on the question being asked. The question may ask about the systemic absorption of different amounts of a topical anesthetic, such as lidocaine, when used to irrigate intubation tubes of respiratory patients. This *if-then* question (*If* different amounts of lidocaine are used, *then* what will the systemic absorption be?) might be answered by designing several experimental groups, utilizing different amounts of lidocaine in differing frequencies, and also using a control group that receives no lidocaine. Systemic absorption of the drug would then need to be measured and compared among the groups. On the other hand, in testing the differences between the readmission rate of diabetic patients who take part in group teaching and those who receive the usual hospital teaching routine, you would need only two groups to answer the question.

In addition to planning the number and type of experimental and control groups, the other major consideration of experimental designs has to do with when and how often the dependent variable will be measured in relation to the occurrence of the independent variable. The dependent variable can be measured before the independent variable is introduced, to establish a baseline, and then measured again after the independent variable has been introduced. This is called a *before-after* design. Here you are looking for a *change* in the dependent variable after the independent variable is introduced. For instance, if you wanted to measure the effect of assertiveness training on subjects in situations where assertive behavior is appropriate, you might measure the response of the subjects to such situations prior to the training program, and again after looking for a change in response that can be attributed to assertiveness training. In this type of design, the subjects are also the controls, since you have their baseline assertiveness to which you can compare future measurements. Some research questions may require several measurements of the dependent variable in order to provide the answer. You may not only be interested in the initial change immediately after assertiveness training, but also in the response after several weeks, so that you can assess the lasting effect of the training.

Some experimental designs only require an *after* measurement of the dependent variable. In this case, the subjects are randomly assigned to experimental and control groups, and no initial measurements are taken. The independent variable is introduced to the experimental group, and then the dependent variable is measured in both groups. In this case, you are looking for a *difference* in the dependent variable between the two groups. For example, if you were testing the effect of a preoperative teaching program on postoperative anxiety, you might use an *after only* design. Subjects would be randomly assigned to the experimental and control groups. Then the independent variable, the teaching program, would be applied to the experimental group. In this case, there is really no way to measure the dependent variable, post-operative anxiety, *before* the introduction of the independent variable. The assumption must be made that because of the random assignment of subjects to the two groups, their *potential* for postoperative anxiety is more-or-less equivalent prior to the teaching program. Therefore, when the dependent variable is measured postoperatively and the two groups compared, the difference in postoperative anxiety can be attributed to the teaching program.

Many research questions in nursing are at a level requiring an experimental design, particularly those that ask about the effectiveness of nursing interventions. If the level of knowledge of the topic is sufficient, and the independent variable is one which can be manipulated, then an experimental design is appropriate.

RECOMMENDED READING

Fisher, R. A. *The Design of Experiments.* Edinburgh: Oliver and Boyd, 1935.

Campbell, D. T., and Stanley, J. C. *Experimental and Quasi-Experimental Designs for Research.* Chicago: Rand McNally, 1963.

Simon, Julian. *Basic Research Methods in Social Sciences.* New York: Random House, 1969.

Strauss, Anselm L., and Glaser, Barney G., *Anguish.* Mill Valley, Calif.: The Sociology Press, 1970.

IX.

Controlling Unwanted Influences

Extraneous Variables
1. Homogeneous Sample
2. Randomization
3. Matching
4. Building Extraneous Variables into the Design

Bias

The Hawthorne Effect

Time

In order to obtain a reliable answer to the research question, the design must show how it proposes to control or eliminate possible alternative answers. The amount of control that the researcher has over the variables being studied varies from a great deal in an experimental design, to very little in an exploratory descriptive design. However, the various unwanted influences that can affect research results must be addressed in any research proposal.

These unwanted influences stem from one or more of the following areas: *extraneous variables, bias,* the *Hawthorne effect,* and the *passage of time.* These four will be discussed in turn, along with some suggestions for controlling their effect. You will have to identify those that seem relevant to your question, and show in your blueprint for action how you will control their effect.

EXTRANEOUS VARIABLES

Extraneous variables are variables that can interfere with the action of those you are studying. They could easily have been chosen as independent variables for your study had you been interested in them, because of their known effect on your variables. Since they are not part of your study, their influence must be controlled.

As an example, a research question asks, "What are the relationships among style of leadership, educational opportunities on the job, and the job satisfaction of staff nurses?" This researcher wonders whether style of leadership and educational opportunities might be having an effect on job satisfaction. However, there are many other factors known to have an effect on job satisfaction. Why not choose age or marital status of the nurse as independent variables? Or the amount of independence on the job, or the level of education of the nurse? Any of these could be independent variables in studying job satisfaction as a dependent variable. But you will choose only those that interest you. The others are all extraneous variables in your study. How can their effect be controlled, so that when the results are tallied, you can actually show the relationship between style of leadership and job satisfaction, and not merely the differences in job satisfaction that are related to the age or educational background of the nurse? Let's look at four different ways of controlling extraneous variables.

Homogeneous sample.   One simple and very effective way of controlling the effect of an extraneous variable on your dependent variable is to eliminate it as a variable from your study; that is, *do not allow it to vary.* Choose a sample that is homogeneous for that variable. For instance, if you are concerned about the effect that the patient's cultural background might have on your study of pain, choose a sample from only one cultural group, such as all Anglo-Saxon Americans, or all Mexican-Americans. You have thereby eliminated any possible effect that the subjects' cultural backgrounds might have on their response to pain, because they all have the same one.

Although effective, this method has one serious drawback: it limits the generalizability of the results. As you might expect, if you study only Mexican-Americans, then your results apply only to Mexican-Americans, and not to blacks, Orientals, or American Indians. If the sample is limited to one age group, the results apply only to that age group, since the relationship you find between your variables might be different for other age groups. You will not know; you can only guess.

Randomization. Theoretically, randomization is the only method of controlling all possible extraneous variables. The random assignment of subjects to the various treatment and control groups means that the groups can be considered *statistically* equal in all ways at the beginning of the experiment. It does not mean that they actually *are* equal for all variables. However, the probability of their being equal is greater than the probability of their not being equal, providing the random assignment was carried out properly. Therefore, we assume that chance is in our favor.

There is tremendous equalizing power in random assignment, except for very small groups. It is a matter of common sense that with very small groups, random assignment could result in unequal distribution of some very crucial variables. If this is likely to be the case in your study, perhaps one of the other methods would be more appropriate. In most instances, however, randomization is the best method of controlling extraneous variables.

Matching. When randomization is not possible, or when the experimental groups are too small and contain some crucial variables, subjects can be matched for those crucial variables. Two subjects are chosen that match each other for the specified variables, such as sex, age, and diagnosis. One of these matched subjects will be assigned to the control group, and the other to the experimental group, thus insuring the equality of the two groups at the onset of the experiment. The process of matching is time-consuming and introduces considerable subjectivity into sample selection. Therefore, it should be avoided whenever possible.

If matching is to be used, keep the number of variables for which the subjects are matched to the smallest possible number. Matching with more than five variables makes it almost impossible to find enough subjects with a matching partner.

Building Extraneous Variables into the Design.   When you cannot adequately control extraneous variables by randomization, they can be built into the design as independent variables. They would have to be added to the purpose of your study and tested for significance along with your other variables. In this way, their effect could be measured and separated from the effect of the variables you wanted to study initially. Particularly in experimental designs, but also in descriptive and explanatory surveys, the effect of these variables can be subtracted statistically from the total action of the variables. This method adds to the cost of the study because of the additional data collection and analysis required. Therefore, it should be used only as a last resort. Other methods should be looked into before this one is chosen.

In exploratory descriptive studies where the nature of the variables is not known, extraneous variables are said to be *built into the design*. The purpose in these studies is to identify the relevant variables and assess their relationship in the data analysis. Therefore, it is essential that you treat all variables as independent during the data collection, so that no data that might later point to relationships between variables will be overlooked. The separation of extraneous variables from independent and dependent variables is part of the analysis of data in exploratory research.

BIAS

Bias results from collecting the data in such a way that one answer to the research question is given undue favor over another. Since bias has to do with the evidence you collect to answer your question, it is a concern during the sample selection and data collection phases of the research process.

All researchers have biased views of their own questions. You know what you want the results to be, and if you are not careful, you will unconsciously sway the study in that direction. Therefore, when you can take precautions to maintain objectivity, you should do so. For example, if you have a choice between randomly selecting your subjects and subjectively picking them out of a group, you should choose random selection. If you plan to interview hospitalized patients, use an available list of patients from which to choose your sample. Do not send an interviewer up to a nursing unit to select patients to interview. That person would probably choose patients who looked like they would enjoy being interviewed, and the sample would most certainly be biased. Another biased sample would result from asking the head nurse to recommend some patients to interview. You would have no idea what criteria were used in making the recommendation, and would not even know the direction of the bias. When random selection is not feasible, make your choice of subjects as objective as possible by reducing the number of choices available to you.

Bias during the data collection means that the researcher is either influencing the responses of the subjects, or is selectively recording observations according to conscious or unconscious predispositions. Both of these problems are present in exploratory studies, especially those where the researcher is involved in the setting with the subjects, such as a nurse collecting data from patients. If data collection is unstructured, and the researcher interacts with the subjects to any great extent, it is virtually impossible to eliminate bias from the study. It is possible, however, to plan for maximum objectivity by building some checks and balances; for example, having an impartial colleague observe with the researcher at least some of the time. Other checks and balances are discussed in the section on reliability and validity in participant observation. You cannot completely eliminate bias from an exploratory study because of the essential flexibility of the design. You can, however, plan for as much objectivity as possible, and keep in mind the limitations of this design when drawing conclusions from your data.

In other types of designs—descriptive survey designs, explanatory survey, and experimental designs—the complete elimination of bias from the data collection becomes more critical. The influence of the investigator's bias on a descriptive response, though difficult to eliminate, can at least be described along with the data. If, however, inferences are to be drawn from the data, there is no room for bias. Therefore, every precaution must be taken to prevent influencing the data collection process in explanatory designs.

THE HAWTHORNE EFFECT

The Hawthorne effect refers to the effect on subjects' responses that result from their knowledge of their status as subjects. In experimental studies, care needs to be taken that the resultant changes in the dependent variable can be attributed to the independent variable and not to the special attention given to the subjects in the experimental group. When testing the effect of nursing interventions, it may be wise to equalize the amount of nursing time spent with patients in both the experimental and control groups, in order to rule out the possibility that the patient is responding to the interaction with the nurse rather than to the intervention. The control group can be thought of as a type of "placebo" group, where nursing interaction is provided without the experimental variable.

In descriptive studies, the Hawthorne effect is created when the presence of an observer affects the behavior of the subjects. The subjects do not behave normally, but rather try to put themselves in a favorable light by assuming what they feel to be more socially acceptable behavior. If the observer is quite unobtrusive, this behavior does not usually last, and the subjects reassume normal behavior after a period of time. The same is true of participant observation once the researcher becomes an accepted member of the group.

TIME

This category is used to cover all those factors resulting from the fact that life goes on during the research process. Events which occur just before or during the study period can affect the responses of subjects, yet have nothing to do with the study; for example, an earthquake, a race riot, or a movie on television. These events can produce changes in attitudes, feelings, and behavior; if the researcher is unaware of their effect, they can lead to erroneous conclusions. To interview patients about sensory disturbances during the aftermath of an earthquake would produce some interesting data. But it would be related to the earthquake rather than to being a patient. If you are questioning people about controversial issues in order to assess their attitudes, it would be wise to check the television schedule for the week of your data collection to avoid coinciding with a special program on your topic.

Developmental or maturational processes also can influence the variables you are planning to measure, particularly if your subjects are very young or very old. This is of special concern when it is necessary to have a long interval between data collection times. The use of control groups may be necessary to rule out the possibility of developmental changes. A special counseling program for minority students, as an example, is expected to ease their adjustment to nursing school. A control group would give substance to the fact that the special counseling program did ease adjustment, and that the students' adjustment was not due simply to the social experience that the school provides.

X.

The Sample

Who Will Be Included?

Methods of Selection
1. Probability Samples
    a. Simple Random Samples
    b. Stratified Random Samples
    c. Cluster Samples

2. Nonprobability Samples
    a. Convenience Samples
    b. Quota Samples

Sample Size

Most research questions contain some reference to the persons, events, or things from which data will be collected to answer the question. This source of data is called the population for the study. The specific composition of the population is defined more clearly in the purpose of the study. In the statement, "The purpose of this study is to describe the stages of the sick role in patients with stroke," the population is *patients with stroke.* When the terms are defined, a further clarification of the population might be, "Patients with stroke are defined as inpatients over 60 years of age, in acute-care hospitals, with newly diagnosed cerebral vascular accidents." This definition provides quite a bit of information about the population, including where to find the subjects. It is unlikely, however, that the researcher plans to study every member of the population, since it is not necessary in order to answer the question. Rather, a *sample* will be selected to represent the population.

A sample is a miniature of a population, and the goal of sampling is to represent the population as closely as possible. Therefore, you must start by clearly defining the population; then you can develop the best way of selecting a representative portion of it. The results of your study are generalized only to the population from which the sample came, provided you can show representation.

WHO WILL BE INCLUDED?

Having defined the population from which the sample will be selected, the next step is to set down some criteria for who will be included in the sample. In the following hypothesis, "There is a significant relationship between the age of the patient and his attitude toward the nurse practitioner," the population is obviously *patients.* In order to test the hypothesis, the patients would have to be those under the care of a nurse practitioner, and would also have to represent different age groups. To set criteria for inclusion in the sample, ask three simple questions: *who, where* and *when?*

QUESTION	ANSWER
Who?	Patients of nurse practitioners. Between 30 and 70 years of age. Able to speak and understand English.
Where?	In the out-patient departments of Kaiser-Permanente Hospitals in the Los Angeles area.
When?	After at least three encounters with a nurse practitioner for diagnosis or treatment.

Answering these three questions about the sample will greatly increase the ease of sample selection. From here you can decide how to select the sample. Let's look at another example:

"The purpose of this study is to determine if there is a difference in the problem-solving abilities of nurses from different educational backgrounds."

QUESTION	ANSWER
Who?	Hospital staff nurses from two-, three-, and four-year programs. Any age, sex, race or ethnic background.
Where?	Working at UCLA Hospital—any unit, shift or specialty area.
When?	Within three years after graduation from nursing school. After six months of employment at UCLA Hospital.

Be as detailed as you can about who qualifies as a subject for your study. It is not necessary to list the criteria for exclusion (who will *not* be included in your study).

When you *replicate* another study, the *who* and *when* questions should be answered the same way as in the original study, but the *where* component might be different. For instance, in the last example, you must use hospital nurses with the same characteristics and amount of experience, but the setting can be different. You might go to U.S.C. Medical Center, or to some other large center similar to UCLA. You might want to use staff nurses from another type of hospital or another part of the country. This element of the sample can be changed, yet the study is still considered a replication.

METHODS OF SELECTION

Once you have set up the criteria for inclusion in your sample, you can determine whether yours will be a *probability* or *nonprobability* sample. In probability sampling, you know that each element in the population has a certain probability of being included in the sample. In nonprobability sampling, there is no way to estimate the probability of each element being included in the sample. Some elements may have no chance at all of being included. The major benefit of probability sampling is that the sample is certain to be representative, making it possible to estimate the degree to which the findings diverge from those that would have been obtained from studying the whole population. In addition, it is possible to calculate the necessary sample size for the margin of error that you are willing to accept. Nonprobability sampling, on the other hand, is usually more convenient and economical. Sometimes nonprobability sampling must be used because no complete listing of the population is available from which to draw a probability sample. Let us discuss both types in further detail.

Probability Samples

The probability sample eliminates the possibility of bias and insures that the sample will be representative. It is based on the availability of a complete listing of all elements in the population from which the sample can be drawn.

Simple Random Samples. The basic probability sampling design is the simple random sample which gives every element in the population an equal chance of being selected. First draw up a numbered list of the population. Then refer to a table of random numbers. Beginning at some arbitrary point on the page, move down the column of random numbers one by one counting off enough to complete your sample size. Now look for numbers from your population list that correspond to the random numbers, and they become your sample. Tables of random numbers can be found in any statistics book and provide the best method of taking simple random samples.

Examples of population lists that can be used by nurses for simple random samples are: members of a state or national nursing organization; all students enrolled at a university; all nurses with a current California state nursing license; all members of the county heart association; all babies born in the county or state during a given day, month, or year; all nursing schools accredited by the National League for Nursing; all hospitals over 200 beds licensed in a given city, or state; all records of patients admitted (or discharged) with a given diagnosis within the last year at a given hospital; all incident reports related to medicine errors within a hospital or series of hospitals. There are many more possibilities; the key element is that a listing be available of all members of the population. Some populations do not have lists available. For instance, if your population is defined as *women in menopause,* you will not find a list of names from any single source. Nor will you find complete listings of populations of heroin addicts, alcoholics, or persons with upper respiratory infections. These populations have no central registry, no gathering place, and unless you redefine your population to include only those receiving some type of treatment, you will have no way to locate a list of the population. This is not to say that you cannot obtain samples of these populations, but rather that the sample cannot be a probability sample and will have to be obtained by some more deliberate method. Keep in mind that the sample must fit the purpose of the study. Therefore your goal must be to find the sample that best represents your population, rather than to obtain one using the most sophisticated sampling technique.

If a simple random sample is both possible and appropriate to your study, there is no better method of selecting subjects. Complete objectivity can be obtained and all bias eliminated, thus strengthening the results of the study.

Stratified Random Samples.   This method is based on the same principle as the simple random sample, except that before the sample is drawn, the population is divided into two or more strata or groups. A simple random sample is then taken from each group. For instance, if having equal numbers of men and women is vital to your study, you can divide the population into two groups according to sex and then draw an equal number of subjects from each.

Note: The variable chosen as a criterion for stratifying a sample must be important to the purpose of the study.

In a study of the effect of educational preparation on nurses' behavior, a stratified random sample might be very appropriate. If a simple random sample of nurses is taken, the proportions of subjects from each type of educational background will not be equal. Therefore, it makes sense to first divide the population into strata according to educational preparation, and then draw equal random samples from each group. The probability of being selected can be calculated for each element in the population, even though it may not be equal among groups.

As with simple random samples, this method requires a complete listing of the population. It also requires information on the criterion for stratification. So if you plan to stratify by educational preparation, your list of the population must include information about educational preparation. The ease with which you can obtain the necessary information about the sample may help make your decision whether to use stratified random sampling. Stratified sampling simply allows you to control the size of the sample from each stratum, and otherwise does not increase the validity of your answer.

Cluster Samples.   In large-scale surveys, when the population represents broad geographic areas or large numbers of people, both simple random samples and stratified samples can be very expensive. A nation-wide sample of nurses might necessitate sending interviewers to scattered localities across the country, and the expense might become prohibitive. A cluster sample would greatly reduce the expense while maintaining the generalizability of probability sampling. The cluster sample method is also called *multi-stage sampling,* because the process of sampling moves through stages until the final sample has been selected.

Starting with the overall population for the study, such as all nursing students in the state, you would proceed as follows:

Prepare a list of counties that have nursing schools and draw a random sample from it. Prepare a list of nursing schools in those counties in the sample and take a random sample of the schools. Then prepare a list of students from these schools and make a random selection of a sample of students. This three-stage process yields a representative sample of nursing students in the state, yet the location of the students is limited first to the counties selected and then to the schools selected from those counties. The savings in time, travel, and expense can be enormous using cluster sampling.

As with simple and stratified random sampling, cluster sampling requires that lists of elements in the population be available. In cluster sampling, however, complete lists are not necessary because of the breakdown into stages.

Nonprobability Samples

The use of nonprobability samples is as often a necessity in nursing research as in other disciplines. Many studies cannot use probability sampling because of the difficulty in obtaining lists of the populations. Experimental designs never use probability sampling because of the need for obtaining informed consent at the beginning of the study. Nonprobability samples are particularly useful with patients when the total population is unknown or not available.

Convenience Samples. A convenience sample is a nonprobability sample that happens to be available at the time of the data collection. To obtain a convenience sample of patients, you could simply plan to include those patients who happened to come into the clinic on data-collection day, or choose the first 50 people who come into the emergency room on a particular Saturday night. There is no way of estimating the potential bias in this kind of sample, but it is possible to plan for objectivity, so that subjects are not deliberately selected by the researcher.

Many samples in nursing studies are convenience samples because of the availability of patient groups through treatment centers. You will probably not know in advance who will come in for treatment and you may have to wait for a sufficient number of new patients to arrive before the sample selection is complete. For instance, if the population is defined as new diabetics being treated for the first time in an out-patient clinic, it may take considerable time for a sufficient number of new diabetic patients to present themselves for diagnosis and treatment at the out-patient department. However, you will estimate approximately how long it will take to obtain your sample, as you know from past information how many patients usually arrive at the clinic each month.

Other examples of convenience samples are: all male Caucasian patients admitted to the CCU for myocardial infarction during the month of February; all mothers of premature infants born during the study period; all children between the ages of two and four who are admitted for tonsillectomy or herniorrhaphy during the study period.

Quota Samples.   As with the convenience sample, the quota sample uses available subjects but takes additional steps to insure inclusion of representatives from all elements in the population. It also attempts to insure that these elements are present in the same proportion in the sample as they appear in the population. This method is used when a convenience sample does not provide the desired balance of elements. For example, the post-partum unit in your hospital may have a patient population that is predominantly Latino; representation of whites and blacks would not appear in sufficient numbers in a convenience sample. In a quota sample, ethnic percentages are specified so that the proportion of each group in the sample represents the ethnic breakdown of total population.

As in stratified random sampling, quota sampling allows you to control the numbers of sample subjects with desired characteristics. When you have several independent variables, for example, age, education, diagnosis, ethnic background, you will have to insure that you have enough subjects in each category of each independent variable so that you have enough data to analyze the relationships among your variables. For example, if you plan to categorize education according to levels in order to analyze the difference between them, you must have a sufficient number of subjects in each category if your analysis is to be valid. In this instance, a quota sample would be appropriate.

SAMPLE SIZE

The best advice for the novice researcher is to use as large a sample as possible. Large samples maximize the possibility that your means, percentages, and other statistics are true estimates of the population. They give the effects of randomness a chance to work. The chance of error goes down in direct proportion to the increased size of the sample. However, practical considerations are important too—for example, how many people are available from your resources?

With random samples, it is possible to set the size of the sample according to how accurately you want to estimate the true population

parameters, or how much "sampling error" you are willing to accept.*
It is possible to devise a number of sampling plans that will insure that
your estimates will not differ from the corresponding true population
figures by, say, more than five per cent (sampling error) on more than
10% of the possible samples that you might draw from the population
(level of confidence). You can also devise plans that will produce
correct results within 2 percentage points, 99 per cent of the time. In
practice, of course, we do not repeat the same study on an indefinite
number of samples drawn from the same population, but it is possible
to predict the probability that the sample will produce data within five
percentage points of that resulting from a study of the whole
population.

If you attempt to predict the necessary sample size for your study
using the formula, you will see that the larger the percentage of
possible error you are willing to accept, the smaller your sample can be.
Therefore, the more accuracy you are trying to achieve, the larger the
sample should be. However, this formula is only applicable to probability samples. When you do use it, you must know the variance of the
measurement you plan to use with your population. This means that
the measurement must be at least at an interval scale, so that the
variance can be calculated. The measurement must also have been
used before with the same or a similar population so that the variance is
known. You will find that if the variance is small, the sample size need
not be as large as when the variance is large. When none of the
measurements vary too far from the mean for the population, it only
takes a small sample to obtain measurements that accurately reflect the
population. But if there is a lot of variation in measurements, a larger
group will be needed to incorporate the entire range of scores in the
sample.

If you know that you can obtain a probability sample, and you
know the variance of the measurement you plan to use, you can decide
on your margin of error and select the optimal sample size to use. But
as mentioned before, there are some practical factors that sometimes
limit your ability to decide on sample size. If you have access to a group
of women undergoing assertion training, and they meet your criteria
for inclusion in your sample, you will probably use the group for your
study, no matter how large or small it may be. The practical factor

---

*The basic formula for computing the sampling error for a sample estimate of
a population parameter is as follows:

$$\text{sampling error} = \frac{\text{variability of the measurement values among the sampling units}}{\sqrt{\text{size of sample}}}$$

influencing your decision is availability. If there is one such group available, take it. If there are many such groups available, then you can plan for the *best* sample size, rather than taking the *available* one.

When you have some choice in planning sample size but cannot use probability sampling, then the size of sample will depend on the number and type of variables that you plan to measure, your goal once again being to insure sufficient data for your analysis. If you plan to look at the relationships between variables, a handy rule-of-thumb is to plan for at least five observations for each category of each variable. If you plot your variables in a chart or table, you can see how many subjects you will need in order to have enough data. For instance, Figure A looks at the relationship between sex, age, and anxiety level. With these variables divided into three categories each, you would need at least 90 subjects. Each variable is then measured once for each subject.

If you plan to measure the same variable many times for the same subject over a period of time, then each measurement can be counted in the same way as you counted subjects in the last example. Look at Figure A again. If anxiety level is to be measured five times for each subject, you will need only one subject for each of the five observations; therefore, the minimum sample size becomes eighteen. In exploratory studies, you will frequently make multiple, in-depth observations of the same subjects, which means that a small sample size will produce a large quantity of data.

Figure A

Relationship among Age, Sex, and Post-Operative Anxiety Level

		MALES			FEMALES		
		20–30	Age 31–40	41–50	20–30	Age 31–40	41–50
ANXIETY LEVEL	Low	5	5	5	5	5	5
	Medium	5	5	5	5	5	5
	High	5	5	5	5	5	5

Total
90

XI.

Selecting a Method to Answer the Question

Observation
1. The Observed and the Observer
2. Methods of Observation

Questionnaires and Interviews
1. Structured Interviews and Questionnaires
2. Unstructured Interviews

Projective Techniques

Available Data

Physiological Measures

The actual method you choose to collect your data depends on several factors. First, it depends on the level of your question, or how much is known about your variables. In an exploratory (Level I) study, you want to amass as much information as possible, and you are not sure just what results to expect. In this case, the best methods are those such as unstructured observation, open-ended interviews and questionnaires, participant observation, and the use of unwritten available data. The advantage of these methods is their flexibility, since you may have to change the questions you ask or the situations you observe as you find out more about the variables.

In a Level II study, where you are looking for relationships between variables, you must have accurate techniques for measuring your variables. Your data must be quantifiable, since you are looking for statistical relationships among the variables. Here, structured observation, questionnaires, and interviews can be used. Written available data and projective tests may be considered. Questions and observations must be comparable from one subject to the next; even open-ended questions must be the same for each subject. The criterion here is accuracy rather than flexibility.

In explanatory (Level III) studies, the investigator controls the situation and the variables. Therefore, the method must be structured. Any method can be used that produces structured, quantifiable data. Conditions and measurements must be identical for all subjects, since inferential statistics will be used to test the hypotheses.

Another consideration in selecting a method is which ones are available and have already been tested and evaluated in measuring your variables. During your search of the literature, some instruments may have come to light that other investigators have developed to measure the variables you are studying. If this is so, by all means use one of these instruments. Using an already-tested instrument provides another link between your study and a growing body of knowledge about your variables. You will be adding to this body of knowledge with your data. But be sure that the instrument fits *your* definition of the variable. Does it measure exactly what you want to know? Only you can decide. Remember that it is possible to adapt an instrument to fit your question, provided you obtain permission from the person who developed it.

If no instruments are available to measure your variables, then you must devise your own. Volumes of material have been written to assist you with this process; you need only decide which method you wish to use and then go to the appropriate source for help. This chapter focuses on some general guidelines to use in devising your own instrument or evaluating one for your study.

OBSERVATION

Observation is a method that we all use every day to collect unstructured data about the world around us. Observation stops being an activity of daily living and becomes a research method when it meets the following criteria: (1) it is systematically planned and recorded; and (2) both observations and recordings are subjected to checks and controls to insure their validity and reliability. These factors make the difference between simply observing the world around you and collecting research data through observation.

Observation is an excellent method of collecting descriptive behavioral data and thus is extremely useful in descriptive studies. It may be the only way to gather some kinds of data. If the information you need cannot be provided by asking the subject questions or through available records, you may have to observe the behavior of the subject and record what you see. Studying the behavior of infants, psychiatric patients, and dying patients; examining the interaction (verbal and nonverbal) between individuals or within groups; looking to see if people behave as they say they will—all these are well suited to the observational method.

Other disciplines also use observational methods; they are not exclusively for the study of human behavior. Chemists collect data on what is observed when two chemicals come in contact with one another. The mating ritual of peacocks is observed and described by biologists; the science of astronomy is almost entirely based on observation and description. Yet in the behavioral sciences, observation is sometimes thought of as a rather unsophisticated method of collecting data.

In nursing, we need to make the most of opportunities to observe and describe patient responses. Even when other methods are used, observations can provide invaluable descriptive material for interpreting the results of the other methods. Therefore, consider, when planning clinical nursing studies, a combination of methods that includes observation.

In planning your observational technique, you will need to consider two basic elements of observation: first, how involved you intend to become with the subjects, and second, how structured you intend your observations to be.

The Observed and the Observer

One dimension of the relationship of the observer and subject is the degree to which the researcher participates in the setting with the subject. Observations collected by nurses in the course of their patient care assignments necessitate their being involved with the patients. Care must be taken to avoid bias in these studies, since it is easy for nurses to influence the responses through subtle changes in their approaches to the patients.

Whether the observer is part of the interaction being studied or simply viewing it, every attempt should be made to keep the interactions as natural as possible. The conspicuousness of the observer in nonparticipant observation is related to the degree of "naturalness" in the subjects' behavior. In this case, the observer should make every effort not to intrude in the situation. The nurse should not be led to believe that her actions are being evaluated or she will not behave naturally. The normalcy of the environment must be maintained.

Methods of Observation

Methods used by observers to collect data can be viewed in terms of the amount of structure they provide. This can range all the way from very unstructured observations, which attempt to provide as complete and nonselective a description as possible, to the very structured method, which attempts to categorize behavior into predetermined categories.

An unstructured observation method might be used to describe the behavior of nurses immediately following the death of a patient. It would involve a complete description of everything the nurse says and does at this time. It should be realized, however, that complete recording of an event is virtually impossible. Even with videotaping, exact replication will not be obtained because of biases introduced by camera angle and lighting. When an observer is attempting a complete recording of an event, some selectivity, both conscious and unconscious, is bound to occur. The observer edits the data according to his or her expectations and biases. This fact should be recognized if you plan to use unstructured observation. As soon as you begin your observations, they will be given structure by your editing process. Even with this editing process, however, a rich depth of material can be gathered from unstructured observation that will never occur using structured methods. As long as the researcher accounts for possible bias in both the data analysis and interpretation, this valuable method can be used to great advantage in nursing research. Of particular value is the combination of unstructured observation with structured methods, which provides more depth to the data.

Structured observation can take one of several forms, but perhaps the most common is the checklist. A checklist allows the researcher to record whether or not a given behavior occurs. The desired behaviors must be explicitly defined so that there is no question in the mind of the observer as to whether or not they occur. For instance, *unhappy* is not a sufficient description. As it stands, the observer would have to interpret observations in light of a personal definition of *unhappy*. A good checklist would specify more operational definitions, such as *visibly crying, refuses treatment, turns back to nurse.* These are all easily-identifiable action definitions. A checklist must be all-inclusive, that is, the researcher must list all of the expected behaviors.

Structured observation, when appropriate, is an excellent method of collecting data. Many more subjects can be observed, in less time, than with unstructured observation, and the data analysis is much simpler. Taking results from a checklist merely involves counting how many times a particular behavior occurred. The results of unstructured observation, on the other hand, consist of quantities of descriptive data, since the observer was trying to record everything that happened. This data must be sorted out to see if there are any patterns to the observed behavior, a very time-consuming process.

You can develop checklists for nursing studies when you know approximately what behaviors to expect. Sometimes a pilot study can be done with a few subjects to give you an idea of the kinds of behaviors to expect. Here a checklist will simplify the data collection. If a checklist is used in exploratory studies be sure to leave space to record unexpected behaviors that are not included in the original list, since your pilot study may not have revealed the entire range of possible behavior.

An example of a checklist used in a nursing study is the following instrument to measure nurses' monitor-watching activity in a Cardiac Care Unit (CCU):

1. Looks at monitor only (at nurses' station).
2. Looks at monitor, goes to bedside, does not talk to patient.
3. Looks at monitor, goes to bedside, talks to patient.
4. Goes to bedside, talks to patient without checking desk monitor.*

This instrument was developed to measure the number of instances in a given time period that CCU nurses behaved in one of the four ways listed above. In this study, the researcher was interested in only those four activities, and therefore had no category for unexpected behaviors.

Since it is usually impossible to observe behaviors for extended periods of time because of fatigue and boredom, you must plan how and when you will make the observations. The two main methods are *time sampling* and *event sampling.*

---

*Adapted from: Irene Stuart, *A Study of the Incidence of Monitor Watching and Nurse-Patient Communication in a Coronary Care Unit,* UCLA Unpublished Masters thesis, 1975.

In *time sampling,* it is customary to divide the day into units that make sense for your observation. For instance, in the previous example of the CCU nurse activities, 15-minute periods make sense since that would allow ample time for a nurse to exhibit any or all of the expected behaviors. One minute would not be sufficient time for one of the behaviors to occur. Several 15-minute periods during an eight-hour shift would provide a good sample of an individual nurse's behavior. The periods can either be randomly selected or predetermined according to the daily routine of the CCU.

Event sampling is used when you need to observe an entire event in order to give the subject the opportunity to perform all of the expected behaviors. If your purpose is to record breaks in sterile technique during dressing changes by student nurses, the sensible approach would be to observe entire dressing change procedures. Time sampling would make no sense at all for this study. Describing nurse-patient interaction during admission to the hospital is another instance when event sampling might be used.

In all of these examples, observation is the best, if not the only way to gather the required data. If you want to know about breaks in sterile technique by student nurses, your alternative method is to ask the student or the patient. Neither of these approaches is likely to produce the data you need. Observation is the best method.

QUESTIONNAIRES AND INTERVIEWS

The preceding discussion emphasized that observational methods are intended primarily to describe behavior as it occurs. Thus, the observable manifestations of the subject's thoughts and emotions provide the data for the study. If you want to know what is *actually* going on inside the subject's head, the easiest way to find out is to ask. Questionnaires and interviews are the two methods designed for this purpose. Because they both rely on verbal reports, they are discussed together. The types of concepts and variables measured by questionnaires and interviews are those having to do with perceptions, attitudes, beliefs, feelings, motives, plans for the future, and events from the past.

The major difference between questionnaires and interviews is the presence of an interviewer in the latter. In questionnaires, responses are limited to answers to the predetermined questions. In interviews, since the interviewer is present with the subject, there is the opportunity to collect nonverbal data as well, and also to clarify the meaning of questions for the subjects if they do not understand.

Using a written questionnaire has some advantages. For one thing, it is likely to be less expensive, particularly in terms of the time spent collecting the data. Questionnaires can be given to large numbers of people simultaneously; they can even be sent by mail. Therefore, it is possible to cover wide geographic areas and to question large numbers of people relatively inexpensively.

Other advantages of questionnaires are that subjects are more likely to feel that they can remain anonymous and thus may be more likely to express controversial opinions. This is more difficult in an interview where the opinion must be given directly to the interviewer. Also, the written question is standard from one subject to the next and is not susceptible to changes in emphasis as can be the case in verbal questioning. There is always the possibility, however, that the written question will be interpreted differently by different readers, which is one of the reasons for careful pretesting of questionnaires.

Interviews have many advantages, the most significant of which is that they can be used to question people who cannot write their responses, for example, patients with eye patches or in traction. This category also includes illiterate subjects, or, as is more frequently the case, subjects who do not write as fluently as they speak. Verbal responses from these individuals will contain much more information than would their written responses.

Another advantage of the interview method is that it usually results in a higher response rate than does the questionnaire. Many people who would ignore a questionnaire are willing to talk with a friendly interviewer who is obviously interested in what they have to say. Hospitalized patients are a good example. Few patients refuse to be interviewed, but questionnaires left at the bedside or given to patients to take home have a much lower response rate.

When conducting an interview, you can be sensitive to misunderstandings by your subjects and provide further clarification if a subject misinterprets a question. In a questionnaire, on the other hand, you will not know whether the subject really misunderstood the question unless the response is quite bizarre. Even then, there is always some doubt as to what to do with such a response.

Another advantage of the interview technique is that you can plan to ask questions at several levels to get the most information from the subject. As an example, the sensory deprivation questionnaires developed by Jackson and O'Neil* start by asking the patient some ambiguous questions, such as, "How have you felt for the last three days?" These are followed by more structured questions, such as, "Did you experience anything out of the ordinary the last three days?" If no reports of sensory disturbances are elicited by these two sets of questions, the interviewer goes on to the very structured questions: "Some-

---

*Jackson, C. Wesley and Margaret O'Neil, "Experiences Associated with Sensory Deprivation Reported for Patients Having Eye Surgery," *Ross Roundtable on Maternal and Child Nursing*, (Columbus: Ross Laboratories, 1966), pp. 54–69.

times people who are in the hospital with conditions like yours do have thoughts, feelings, and experiences which they wonder about. For example, they see things and wonder if they are real. If anything like this happened to you the last three days, would you describe it for me?" This approach is unique to the interview. The combination of structured and unstructured questions can provide depth and richness to the data, and at the same time, elicit data that are comparable from one subject to the next.

When looking for a questionnaire or interview schedule to use in your study, or when developing your own tool, you will have to consider the various kinds of questions that you can ask to obtain a range of data, and then decide which method is best suited to your variables. The content of the questions must be considered first, and then the amount of structure in the format.

Question content, or the purpose of the question, falls into two basic categories: those aimed at getting facts from the subject, and those aimed at getting the subject's perception or feelings. Factual questions ask subjects for information either about themselves, or about events or people about which they have reason to know something. Questions asking for demographic data (age, marital status, income, education, etc.) fall into this category. So do questions asking the individual to recall an event or sequence of events ("Tell me about the events leading to your coming to the hospital.")

Nonfactual questions deal with the subjects' perception of what happened or their feelings about people, events, or things. They may also deal with the subjects' reasons for their behavior ("Why did you call the doctor at that particular time?"). In these kinds of questions, you are not interested in whether the subject's report is accurate but rather in the subject's *perception,* which may or may not accurately reflect the facts.

The format of interviews and questionnaires, as with observational methods, can range from very structured to very unstructured, depending on how much is known about the range of possible responses.

Structured Interviews and Questionnaires

Structured questionnaires are standardized tests in which the questions are presented in exactly the same way, with the same wording, and in the same order to all the subjects. Standardizing the questions insures that all the subjects are responding to the same question so that the responses can be compared. The order of the questions may affect how the subject will answer; therefore, standardized questions are always given in the same order to all subjects.

The most structured questions are *fixed alternative* questions in which the subject is asked to choose one of the given alternatives. Some examples of fixed alternative questions are as follows:

(i)   Check the response that best describes how you feel about each statement:

"Alcoholism is basically a character disorder."

Strongly agree _ Agree _ Neutral _ Disagree _ Strongly disagree_

(ii)   Which of the following is your choice of specialty area? Choose only one.

_____ 1. Medical or Medical Intensive Care
_____ 2. Surgical or Surgical Intensive Care
_____ 3. Obstetrics: Labor and Delivery, Postpartum or Newborn Nursery, and specialties within these areas
_____ 4. Pediatrics and area specialties
_____ 5. Psychiatric and area specialties

(iii)   Which three of the following life events have been most difficult for you? Please rank your three choices in order from the most difficult (1) to least difficult (3).

_____ 1. Childhood
_____ 2. Marriage
_____ 3. Retirement
_____ 4. Illness of self or spouse
_____ 5. Death of spouse or other close relative
_____ 6. Children left home
_____ 7. Parenthood

Questions such as these are the same whether used in a questionnaire or an interview. They are more commonly used in questionnaires but may be used in interviews, particularly if the subject is unable or unwilling to fill out a questionnaire.

Open-ended questions are less structured than the fixed-alternative kind and give subjects more leeway to provide their own answers. The question is designed to allow the subject a free response, rather than a response limited or guided by given alternatives. Some examples of open-ended questions are as follows:

(i) How do you feel about abortions?

(ii) What do you think women should do to ensure equal rights?

(iii) What do you dislike most about heroin addicts?

These questions can also be used in both interviews and questionnaires. In interviews, probing questions can be used with them as follow-ups if the subject does not volunteer enough information in response to the open-ended question. These might be, "Won't you tell me more?" or "What makes you say that?" However, with the use of probing questions, the interview moves from the category of structured questions to unstructured interviews.

Unstructured Interviews

In exploratory research, it may not be appropriate to structure the interview questions in advance, other than to decide on your opening statement or question. A flexible interview, when properly used, can bring out much useful material because it allows the interviewer to pursue whatever avenue seems important to the subjects, and thus can elicit the subjects' values, beliefs, and attitudes. Their responses will be completely spontaneous, self-revealing, and personal.

The flexibility of the interview is both an advantage and a disadvantage to the researcher. The results will not be comparable from one subject to the next because the interview format is never the same. However, it is invaluable in exploring the whole range of attitudes, thoughts, and feelings that exist for the topics.

Sometimes the interview has a focus, as in psychiatric evaluations where the interviewers have a list of topics to cover but can select their own method of eliciting the information. Also left up to the interviewer is whether to pursue an avenue that seems of particular interest.

Another unstructured interview uses the *nondirective* technique. Here the initiative is almost completely in the hands of the subject. The interviewer's function is to encourage the subject to talk but with a minimum of guidance. The main function of the interviewer is to show interest in the subject and anything the subject cares to talk about, thus serving as a catalyst for the expression of the subject's feelings. This type of interview requires considerable skill on the part of the interviewer.

The interview and questionnaire are tools used by every nurse in patient care—the patient's self-report is one of our most valuable data collection methods. Although nurses are more accustomed to the interview technique, they also see the value of questionnaires. The important thing to remember when choosing a method is that it be the most appropriate one for measuring the variables *as you have defined them.*

Whether you use the interview or questionnaire method, it must be because your operational definition calls for the subject's *self-report*. If it does not, or if there is reason to believe that the person cannot give a valid response (for example, you may be trying to measure an unconscious process), then these methods are not appropriate and you must choose another.

PROJECTIVE TECHNIQUES

There are times when the variables you are trying to measure are neither observable nor obtainable from the subject because they represent feelings or attitudes that the individual is unable or unwilling to report. *Projective techniques* are indirect methods of measuring these variables. They typically involve some type of imaginative activity on the part of the subject in response to an ambiguous stimulus. The use of these techniques requires intensive specialized training beyond the scope of most nurses. However, some nurses will have this training and others will have access to people who do, making some discussion of projective techniques appropriate.

The stimuli used in a projective test must be capable of arousing many different kinds of reactions; for instance, an inkblot that can appear to be many different things; a picture that can elicit many different stories; toys that can be used to portray many people and events. The subject's perception of the stimulus, the feelings it arouses, and the way the subject organizes these responses, provide the data for analysis by the expert. The responses are not taken at face value but instead are interpreted according to predetermined conceptualizations.

The *Rorschach Inkblot Test* consists of ten cards, each of which depicts an inkblot. The subject is shown each card and asked, "What might this be?" The *Thematic Apperception Test* (TAT) provides a series of pictures about which the subject is asked to tell stories. Both of these frequently-used techniques are designed to elicit a rich sample of responses from which a wide variety of inferences can be drawn. Other commonly-used projective tests are *word association, sentence completion,* and *figure drawing.*

Projective tests all rely on the fact that people often find it easier to be expressive when they are not talking specifically about themselves and their own feelings. Talking through the medium of the projective test allows the subjects to maintain a distance from their own thoughts and feelings, enabling them to talk impersonally about themselves. In addition, feelings of which the subject may not be consciously aware appear in the responses to the ambiguous stimulus.

If your operational definition calls for a projective measure, you will want to consider one of the approaches we have discussed. Keep in mind, however, that most projective measures require the assistance of an expert to analyze the subjects' responses. If this is not available to you, you may have to abandon this method of data collection, even though it might be the most suitable.

AVAILABLE DATA

The health field offers a multitude of available data. Using this type of data is certainly economical. It has other advantages as well. Most official records have been collected over time, thus making it possible to follow trends. Time and money are saved by the availability of a large sample of records in one location.

The kind of available data that comes to mind for nursing research is the medical record. Hospitals keep medical records on hand for at least five years, and have records dating back much further that are retrievable for research purposes. Also available through hospital records departments are admission rates by age, sex, diagnosis, and other variables. They also have data on length of stay, types of surgeries performed, and so on. Much information about work patterns of nurses can be found in personnel records, and in the records of staffing patterns kept by nursing departments.

Data from entire communities can be found in census records and in records from public health departments. These can be used to look for trends within a community, or to compare one community with another.

Less frequently, data from newspapers, magazines, professional journals, textbooks and the like are used for research purposes. In historical studies, personal documents such as autobiographies, letters, and diaries can provide a wealth of data. Mass communications can also provide useful information. For instance, consider the possibility of analyzing the image of the nurse as presented on television or in movies.

Unwritten sources of available data include television, motion pictures, tape recordings, photographs, and in rare cases, an historian studying a culture without written records. The use of historical artifacts, buildings, architecture, clothing and the like are examples of unwritten available data, and are possible sources of data for nursing studies.

The major drawback in using available data, no matter how they were collected, is that they were not compiled primarily for your study and, therefore, may not quite fit with your definition of terms. For instance, if you were collecting data on the number of times patients are transferred from room to room during their hospital stay, you might go to the hospital daily census as a source only to discover that this document only lists transfers from one nursing unit to another and not those made from room to room within the same unit. Hopefully, this is something you would find out before you began to collect data, but sometimes there is no way of knowing how the data were collected and how the recorders defined the categories of data. You can, therefore, obtain misleading results using available data.

For instance, suppose you wanted to compare the nurse-patient ratio among several hospitals in your area. Each hospital has data available that can be translated into a nurse-patient ratio. However, you might find that one hospital that appears to have fewer patients per nurse actually includes head nurses and unit secretaries in its staffing figures, whereas other hospitals do not. If you are not aware of how the data are reported, you might be misled by your findings.

When using nurses' notes as a source of data, you must take into account the fact that the nurses doing the recording had no common operational definitions for the terms they used. Even simple terms like "slept well" have different meanings for different nurses. An operational definition established for research purposes has to specify exactly what is meant by "slept well," and how it is to be differentiated from "slept poorly" or other categories. Thus "slept well" might become "when checked every half hour during the hours of midnight to 6 a.m., the patient was asleep." When operational definitions are not available, the individual data collectors use their own definitions. As long as this fact is taken into account, much valuable information can be found in nurses' notes and other such records.

PHYSIOLOGICAL MEASURES

As a method of data collection, nurses have the opportunity to utilize a wealth of physiological measures. These provide objective data relating to patients' responses to nursing care and should not be overlooked as sources of valuable data. Physiological methods can be used alone or in conjunction with other methods. They can be used as the data collection method for your study, or the results of physiological measures can be obtained from available records, such as patients' charts.

Physiological measures available to nurses range from simple ones such as blood pressure, pulse, and temperature to the measurement of sodium and potassium ratios in 12-hour urine collections as an indicator of stress. Nurses can use measurements such as tidal volume and blood gases to measure the response to treatment of respiratory patients. In a study of the physiological effects of shift rotation on ICU nurses, Tooraen used the measurement of 17-hydroxycorticosteroids as an index of overall adrenal cortical secretory activity, but rather than measuring it directly, measured increases in sodium and potassium in the urine.*

With the complex monitoring equipment available in all critical care units, nurses have the opportunity to study many variables that formerly could not be accurately measured. Instant and continuous measures of physiological response can be obtained for patients in critical care units. In addition, such equipment can be obtained through schools of nursing and medical centers for research with healthy subjects.

RECOMMENDED READING

Dunn, Margaret A. "Development of an Instrument to Measure Nursing Performance," *Nursing Research*. 19:502–510, November–December, 1970.

Payne, Stanley L. *The Art of Asking Questions*. Princeton, N.J.: Princeton University Press, 1951.

Rich, Rosemary and James K. Dent. "Patient Rating Scale," *Nursing Research*. 11:163–171, Summer, 1962.

Moreno, J. L. (ed.) *Sociometry and the Science of Man*. New York: Beacon House, 1956.

Oppenheim, A. N. *Questionnaire Design and Attitude Measurement*. New York: Basic Books, 1966.

Pigors, Paul and Faith Pigors. "The Incident Process—A Method of Inquiry," *Nursing Outlook*. 14:48–50, October, 1966.

Osgood, Charles E. and James G. Snider. *Semantic Differential Technique: A Sourcebook*. Chicago: Aldine Publishing Co., 1969.

Webb, Eugene J., Donald Campbell, Richard Schwartz and Lee Sechrest. *Unobtrusive Measures: Nonreactive Research in the Social Sciences*. Chicago: Rand McNally, 1966.

Smith, Patricia Cain, Lorne M. Kendall and Charles L. Hulin. *The Measurement of Satisfaction in Work and Retirement*. Chicago: Rand McNally, 1969.

---

*Sister Lynda Ann Tooraen, "Physiological Effects of Shift Rotation on ICU Nurses," *Nursing Research* 21, No. 5 (Sept–Oct 1972): 398–405.

XII.

Reliability and Validity of Measurement

Reliability
1. Test-retest
2. Repeated Observations
3. Equivalence
4. Alternate Forms
5. Split-Half Method

Reliability and Validity of Participant Observation
In Exploratory Studies
Validity
1. Face Validity
2. Construct Validity
3. Content Validity
4. Concurrent Validity
5. Predictive Validity
Reliability
1. Test-retest
2. Repeated Observations
3. Equivalence

Some Conclusions on Validity and Reliability

The quality of your research results depends first on your ability to develop a clear and logical research problem from your initial question, then on the ability of your research design to produce an adequate answer to your question. The adequacy of the research design depends on the quality of the measurement procedures themselves—their validity and reliability. The answer to the question is based on the data collected by these procedures; therefore, the answer is only as good as the procedures.

The operational definitions include your definition of the variable and how you intend to measure it—observation; a questionnaire or interview; physiological measures; or available data. Whichever technique you have decided to use, it must produce information that is not only relevant to your research question, but also *accurate*. The two aspects of accuracy that must be addressed in the research proposal are *reliability* (the extent to which the measure gives consistent results), and *validity* (the extent to which the measurement reflects the subject's true relation to the characteristic being measured).

A measurement procedure is considered reliable when a series of measurements give similar results. A yardstick, for example, is a highly reliable instrument. An object can be measured daily, and unless it changes in size, it will measure exactly the same each day. On the other hand, an intelligence test is considered unreliable if a person scores very high at one test period and very low at another time, when nothing has happened which might explain such a change.

But consistent results may not be valid ones. Repeated measurements of the same object with a poorly-calibrated ruler would yield the same results but would not be a valid measure of the object's length. A tool developed to measure attitudes toward abortion might produce consistent results but actually be measuring strength of religious beliefs.

In addition to being valid and reliable, a research instrument should be *sensitive*, that is, capable of making fine-enough distinctions. For example, an instrument measuring attitudes toward abortion might be a very crude instrument measuring only two positions; *for* and *against*. A more finely-graduated instrument would provide several varying degrees of these positions. It is then more "sensitive" and can pick up smaller differences in attitudes.

VARIATIONS IN SCORES

Measurement results reflect not only the true differences in the characteristic being measured, but also other unknown factors that affect both the characteristic being measured and the measurement process. Here are some possible sources of differences in scores.

True Differences.   Ideally, all of the differences in scores among individuals would be due to differences in the characteristic being measured. For instance, if a questionnaire is supposed to measure depression, all of the differences in scores among the sample would reflect the individuals' differing levels of depression. None would reflect chance variations or the effects of other attitudes or characteristics. The perfect instrument, one that meets these criteria, does not exist. Our goal is to reduce the effect of other sources of differences so that the instrument approaches the ideal as nearly as possible.

Stable Personal Factors.   Many personal variables can influence scores: intelligence, education, social status, personality characteristics. Two in particular have been frequently found to affect the measurement of other characteristics. These are the tendency to give a favorable impression of one's self, and the tendency to agree (or disagree) with statements regardless of their content. Both affect responses to questionnaires and interviews. Measurements that ask for responses to statements that might be influenced by social desirability. It has been demonstrated that some people tend to agree or disagree with series of statements regardless of their content, apparently a relatively stable characteristic of these individuals. It is recommended that researchers attempt to rule out the most likely contaminating variables as sources of variance in scores.

Transient Personal Factors.   Mood, fatigue, state of health, attention span: these are personal factors that can vary even within a short period of time. It has been suggested that the pervasiveness of these transient personal factors is related to motivation. Under proper conditions of motivation, their effect is negligible. Motivation is highest when the topic of the questionnaire or interview interests the respondent.

Situational Factors.   Environmental factors such as light, heat, and comfort can create differences in an individual's responses to measuring instruments. So can the degree of anonymity provided by the situation—the presence or absence of other people (a family member or roommate) in an interview.

Variations in Administration.   Inadequate and nonuniform methods of administering an instrument may contribute to variations in scores. Interviewers may change words, add instructions, or omit questions so that one interview is not comparable with another. Bored test administrators may improvise their own instructions. A tired observer may not notice that the atmosphere of the group has changed. All of these variations in the use of the instrument may markedly affect the consistency of the data obtained.

Lack of Clarity of the Instrument. If individuals understand the questions differently, their responses may reflect these differences in interpretation rather than true differences in the characteristic you are trying to measure. Take the question, "Do you have good relations here at work?" Three responses of *No* could mean: No, I can't stand anyone here; No, I would never work with anyone in my family; No, I never indulge in personal relations on the job.

In addition to these sources of difference are the errors that can be made in scoring and totaling the scores, tabulation, machine analysis, or statistical computations. Thus, there are many sources of error in measurement of variables that can influence the results. These sources of error can be classified as constant (systematic, biasing) or random (variable). A constant error is one that systematically affects the characteristic being measured or the process of measurement, for example, stable personal factors. Random error results from the subject's transient aspects, which may vary from one time of measurement to the next. Random error shows up in the consistency of repeated measurements for the same subject. Estimates of validity are concerned with both constant and random errors; estimates of reliability usually take into account random errors only.

VALIDITY

With any instrument, ask the question, "What does it measure?" The validity of an instrument is defined as the extent to which it measures what it is intended to measure, without being affected by constant or random error. No instrument measuring characteristics of human behavior is completely valid. For any single instrument we try to increase its validity by eliminating, as much as possible, its susceptibility to other influences. Since such influences can never be completely eliminated, two or more measures should be used whenever possible that differ in the particular extraneous influences that affect it. The importance of validity cannot be overemphasized. An answer based on invalid data is of no value to you or anyone else. It may provide grossly misleading results and seriously hamper the development of knowledge about your topic.

Concurrent and Predictive Validity. Both are pragmatic approaches, the interest being in judging the instrument's usefulness as an indicator or a predictor of a specific behavior or characteristic. With a pragmatic approach, you ask questions of the tool such as, "Does it work?" "Does it help to distinguish individuals with regard to some criterion?" A tool that helps to distinguish people according to their present status is said to have *concurrent validity*. For instance, it may distinguish between children who are mentally retarded and those who are developing normally. A test that can be used now to predict an event that will occur in the future is said to have *predictive validity*. The researcher might develop an entrance exam for nursing students that would predict who would pass State Board exams. The essential ingredient in this approach to validation is a reasonably valid and reliable criterion with which the scores on the instrument can be compared.

Construct Validity. Most often, we are interested in measurements as a basis for inferring the degree to which the individual possesses some characteristic or trait (alienation, intelligence, attitude toward illness, depression, anxiety, etc.). This characteristic or trait presumed to be reflected in the score is not a specific action, but rather an abstraction or construct. The process of validating this kind of measuring instrument is called *construct validation*. The researcher generally starts with the factors thought to explain the variance of the test; these come from the theory upon which the test is based. In an intelligence tests, these factors might be verbal ability, abstract reasoning ability, and social class membership. Other measures of these variables can be correlated with the score from the intelligence test to provide a measure of construct validity. At the same time, the theory underlying the instrument is being tested.

Self-evident Measures. Observations of behavior for descriptive purposes are said to have *face validity*. That is, the relevance of the instrument to the variable being measured is self-evident. For example, reading speed is measured by computing how much a person reads with comprehension in a given time. Job performance might be rated according to the quality and quantity of work produced. *Content validity*, the degree to which the content of the instrument is representative of what is known about the topic, can be estimated from the literature or by a panel of experts.

RELIABILITY

As pointed out earlier, scores on measuring instruments reflect not only the characteristic the instrument is intended to measure, but also a variety of other influences, some constant and some transitory. The evaluation of an instrument's reliability consists of estimating how much of the variation in scores is due to transitory influences (random errors). The less the scores are influenced by such factors, the more reliable is the instrument. If we know an instrument is valid, we need not worry about its reliability—a valid instrument measures accurately. However, unless satisfactory validity or reliability has already been demonstrated, an instrument should be tested for reliability before it is used in a study, rather than after. The following are methods of estimating the reliability of an instrument.

Test-retest. The identical interview may be given to the same individuals at different times under equivalent conditions, and the results of the two measurements can be compared. The same can be done with questionnaires or other tests. However, it must be remembered that the very process of remeasurement may intensify differences in transient factors; for example, anxiety, interest, and motivation may be lower during the second testing. Moreover, the subjects may remember the responses they gave to the first test (particularly if the time interval is short) and give these remembered responses rather than thinking through the question again. There is the further possibility that the first test may raise the subject's interest in the subject and lead to increased knowledge or a change in attitudes before the second testing. Then, of course, there is the possibility of a permanent genuine change between the two testings. Therefore, the common practice is to try to wait long enough for the effects of the first testing to wear off but not long enough for a significant change to occur. It is better to wait too long and obtain an underestimate of reliability than not long enough and be mislead by the resulting overestimate.

Repeated Observations. This approach is similar to the test-retest, and is used when the measuring instrument consists of observations. Supposing you were interested in the percentage of time a CCU nurse spends in monitor-watching, as compared to all other activities. You could randomly select a fifteen-minute period while the nurse is on duty, and record the amount of time spent in monitor-watching. From this record, you could easily calculate the percentage of time spent monitor-watching. After repeating this process several times, you will have a series of percentages representing the proportion of time the nurse spent watching the monitor according to your observations. You can then look at the range of percentages, their standard deviation, or some other measure of their variability to see how stable they are. Note that both test-retest and repeated observations can only be done when the characteristic you are measuring is relatively stable.

Equivalence. In the example of the CCU nurse, we assumed a single observer who was responsible for all the measurements made. But what if this observer were biased or careless? You can eliminate this possibility by having different observers who have been trained in the same way watch the same nurse simultaneously and independently record their observations. Any discrepancies that emerge can be clarified, or the procedure repeated, until the observations are more or less equivalent.

Alternate Forms.   In this procedure, supposedly equivalent forms of the same test are given to the same individuals at the same testing session. Although the two forms contain different items, the items are intended to measure the same thing. The correlation between scores on the two forms indicates the extent to which they are actually measuring the same characteristic in a consistent fashion. This method eliminates the problem of random changes occuring over time. However, it is often a cumbersome procedure. For one thing, it is hard to develop two equivalent tests. Also, the test period for the subjects is doubled, which may affect their response. For this reason, the subjects are usually divided in half. One form is given first to one half; the other, to the other half. This still does not eliminate the possibility of fatigue and annoyance at being asked the same question in a slightly different way. Alternate forms are probably most useful when the research design calls for repeated measurements of the same subjects. In this case, the tests should differ enough in specific content to lessen the possible effects of memory, but be alike enough so that the results can be compared.

Split-half Method.   When alternate forms are not required or are difficult to achieve, a split-half correlation may be used that incorporates both forms into a single test. In this procedure, a single form of a test is given once to a group of subjects. The items on the test are then divided into two halves and the scores on the two halves are correlated to estimate their equivalence. The assumption is that a person will respond in the same way to one half of the items as the other half. The usual way of dividing the items is to compare odd-numbered items with even-numbered items. A correlation is done and corrected split-half reliability calculated using the Spearman-Brown formula.* Although this method is used extensively, current thinking is that if all items in the test are intended to measure the same characteristic, random rather than equivalent halves should be compared. Formulas have been developed (Kuder-Richardson 20) that give the average split-half correlation for all possible ways of dividing the test into two parts and thus satisfy the requirement for randomness.

$$*R_{sp-bn} = \frac{2(r)}{1 + r}$$

RELIABILITY AND VALIDITY OF PARTICIPANT OBSERVATION IN EXPLORATORY STUDIES

In exploratory studies that use participant observation as the method of data collection, the researcher becomes part of the group being studied, and moves from stranger to familiar. Since strangers cannot distinguish leaders from followers, nor make a basic differentiation of who's who in the group in relation to age, sex, social status, and social ranking, it is necessary to become familiar with the group in order to learn these things. However, because the researcher remains basically a stranger, all data are subject to bias, distortion, and gross error. Therefore, the methods used to minimize error requires some discussion.

In order to put exploratory studies into perspective with other designs, the following discussion on reliability and validity uses the same terminology as was used to discuss the reliability and validity of instruments, even though these terms were not developed for the exploratory study. The difficulty lies in the fact that the participant-observer is the major research instrument, and the major source of data is the informant, both of whom are human beings—notoriously unreliable, sometimes unethical, always biased. Nevertheless, an attempt must be made to ascertain the reliability and validity of the source and the instrument, since the value of the results hinges on both.

Validity

Face Validity. On the assumption that all members of a culture are carriers of that culture, any person who belongs to the group under study is a possible informant. That is, each member of the population has *face validity*. The researcher as observer is also assumed to have face validity. For instance, in a study of heroin addicts in a live-in treatment center, if participant observation is to be the method, it is assumed at the beginning of the project that any addict who is a member of the group has face validity as an informer, and the researcher, even though a stranger to the group, has face validity as an observer.

Construct Validity. The degree to which members of a group possess a particular cultural trait or status is established by the informant's statement in conjunction with the statements of others. Frequently, informants want to impress the researcher with their own importance in the group, and therefore accord themselves higher status or a more important role in the group than they actually possess. Validation of status and role is accomplished by questioning someone other than a close friend or relative of the informant—an uninterested party or even an enemy of the informant.

Construct validity is always used for ascertaining degrees of differences between individuals and groups, whether the differences are due to age, sex, experience, education, or election. And always, the most intimately involved are used as primary informants and uninterested parties used for confirmation.

Content Validity.   Since informants must be qualified to discuss their cultural knowledge, clarification of their status and roles in relation to the subject matter must be made. Men are not viable informants on women's secrets, nor women for men's. Using them as such would provide hearsay evidence and not full insider knowledge. First-offender addicts cannot serve as sources for information about repeaters, nor can those at the center of their own volition give valid information about those who were sentenced to treatment by the court. In addition, the investigator must learn the social position of the informant prior to accepting the interview as valid. More than one informant is used for any single element in order to cross-check the collected data. Each informant is considered to be an expert on a particular content area and at least two expert informants are used with each content area to establish validity.

Content validity is established for observations through the use of a panel of expert informants, who are asked to certify that the event, behavioral sequence, or situation is representative of the situation being observed. Each group of addicts within the treatment center may have modifications for particular behaviors; therefore informants from the group in which the event occurs are required to establish the norms of that group. Cross-checking informants' statements within and across groups will establish norms for one group and for the population as a whole.

Concurrent Validity.   The major method of establishing concurrent validity in participant observation is the use of interviews in conjunction with observations. Here the researcher is comparing what informants says they do against what is actually done in the situation.

Another method is for the investigator to have another observer along when observing an event. The researcher observes status symbols, deference behaviors, who talks to whom, the nature of the interactions, and so on. To validate these observations, the second observer is asked *during* the event to validate impressions. At the same time, information to further clarify relationships between participants in the event can be obtained. This form of concurrent validity is extremely important for events that the researcher does not anticipate seeing again.

Predictive Validity.   Closely related to concurrent validity, predictive validity also relies on the combination of interviews and observations. In the course of an interview, the informant explains, describes, and predicts what will happen in any given situation. The informant may be describing his or her own behavior, behavior of others, or the behavior of the group as whole. The researcher can then validate that prediction with his or her own observations. Any deviations from the prediction, major or minor, are later clarified with the informant.

Reliability

Since establishing validity obviates the need for establishing reliability, little work is left once validity is established. However, there are times when validity cannot be established for participant observation, requiring testing for reliability.

Test-retest.   Every major informant is subjected to more than one interview over time in which the same questions are repeated. The answers to the questions can be treated as a test-retest, and changes or discrepancies noted. In this way, a measure of the reliability of an individual informant can be estimated.

Repeated Observations.   Many behaviors, events, and situations will occur frequently enough during the course of the study that the observer becomes completely familiar with them. By taking advantage of these opportunities to record repeated observations, the researcher establishes a measure of his or her own reliability as an observer. Greetings, etiquette, and eating habits are examples of repetitive events that can be used as repeated observations.

Equivalence.   Whenever possible, researchers uses informants or other researchers to observe an event or behavior along with them. Each independently records his or her own observations, which are compared following the event. Interviews can be treated similarly. The purpose is to determine if the content of the observation or interview was the same for both persons who were recording it. Discrepancies can then be clarified, or the procedure repeated until both parties observe the same event similarly. As with repeated observations, this method provides an estimate of the reliability of the researcher as an observer.

SOME CONCLUSIONS ON VALIDITY AND RELIABILITY

Since exploratory research requires an inordinate amount of explanation, most reports of participant observation do not deal with the methods used to establish the reliability and validity of the data collection. Therefore, the novice researcher might get the impression that these areas are neglected in exploratory research. In explanatory studies, on the other hand, there is a tendency to overemphasize the reliability and validity of the instrument in the research report, sometimes giving the impression that little else was accomplished by the study. Neither emphasis is appropriate, since the usability of the research depends on complete reporting of both the findings and the methodology.

The proposal, which is the subject of this book, requires *complete reporting* of the methods to be used to establish reliability and validity. The proposal is not subject to the whims and fancies of editors and publishers; therefore, adequate time and space can be given to a discussion of the validity and reliability of your instruments. If you are developing your own instrument, you must show your plans for a pilot study to test and revise the instrument until it is accurate enough to use in your study.* If you are using an available instrument, you must describe how its reliability and validity were tested, and show how you plan to further establish the instrument for use with your sample.

When using an available instrument, it may not be necessary to do a pilot study, particularly if the instrument has been used before with a sample similar to yours. But if you have changed the instrument at all to adapt it to your study, then you must retest for reliability.

When doing a replication study, the reliability and validity of the instrument must be re-established. The method does not have to be exactly the same as the original study, but it may not be a lower level method than the original study used. In other words, it is acceptable to provide more information than the original author did, but never less.

RECOMMENDED READING

Cronbach, L. and P. Meehl. "Construct Validity in Psychological Tests," *Psychological Bulletin*. 52:281–302, 1955.

Fiske, D. and P. Pearson. "Theory and Techniques of Personality Measurement," *Annual Review of Psychology*. 21:49–86, 1970.

---

*A correlation of .8, using the split-half, test-retest, or alternative form methods, is considered adequate for general use.

XIII.

Protection of Human Rights

2. Resources for Decision Making
   a. Colleagues
   b. Consultants
   c. Committees for the Protection of Human Subjects

Maintaining Anonymity and Confidentiality
1. Plan Ahead
2. Data Banks
3. Legal Problems
4. Publication

What happens to those who take part in research? Who is concerned with their welfare? These questions received little attention from researchers until recent years. In the past, researchers have not only involved their subjects in research without permission, but also gave false information about the role of the subject in the study and involved people in experiments that were harmful both physically and psychologically. Little attention was paid to the rights of the subjects; the all-important factor was the scientific contribution of the research.

Today, it is of utmost importance to researchers in all disciplines that the rights of subjects be protected to the fullest possible extent. When the subjects are vulnerable, as is true of patients, the researcher's proposal must explain how their rights will be protected.

Not only are the researchers themselves concerned with the subjects, government agencies and legislatures at the state and federal level are also concerned with invasion of privacy and experimentation with human subjects. In 1974, Congress established a National Commission for Protection of Human Subjects of Biomedical and Behavioral Research. This commission recommends legislative and regulatory action to govern agencies issuing research grants.

As clinical nurses become more involved in research, the issue of protection of human rights becomes a critical one. This is primarily because of the ease with which nurses can collect data for research as part of their practice, with or without the knowledge or consent of the patient. The profession must assume the responsibility for ethical practices in nursing research.

Although the discussion of protection of human rights more appropriately belongs with the sample, it involves many issues that arise at various times during the planning process. Therefore, an entire chapter is devoted to this topic.

INFORMED CONSENT

Just as all patients entering the health care system have the right to informed consent for any and all aspects of their care, so does the participant in research have this same right. The whole subject of protection of human rights revolves around obtaining a true informed consent from the subjects.

What is informed consent? Informed consent includes knowledge about the nature, duration, and purpose of the study; the methods and procedures by which data will be collected and how it will be used; all inconveniences and potential harm or discomfort that might reasonably be expected; and the results, effects, and side effects that may come from participation in the study. The rights of the research subject include the right to stop participating at any time during the study and to expect the data to remain confidential.

Obviously, not all research meets the criteria for informed consent. Many studies fail in one or more of these areas to completely protect the subjects' rights, often because complete informed consent is impossible. The reasons vary from using data from deceased subjects to giving subjects incomplete or incorrect information so as not to bias the data. Whatever the reason, however sound, just, and reasonable it may be, all violations of the basic right of subjects to informed consent result in ethical problems for the researcher. These problems must be attacked in the proposal and may be so pervasive that the researcher must consider abandoning the study.

PROBLEMS INVOLVING ETHICS

No Consent

In the past, many significant studies were carried out in which the subjects never knew that they had participated in a research project. Sometimes it was impossible or impractical to tell them. Sometimes the researcher decided that such knowledge would create unnatural behavior and distort the research results. Whatever the excuse, the result is a violation of the subjects' right to decide whether or not to participate. Whenever possible, ways to avoid involuntary participation must be sought, and if there are truly none, then the benefits of the research must be carefully weighed against the ethical costs.

In nursing research this issue arises in many types of studies. These include observational studies of patient or nurse behavior and studies where data are collected as part of the researcher's normal professional activities.

Observational Studies. These studies may employ participant or nonparticipant observation; in either case, the subjects are not informed of the study. An example is the observation of the behavior of patients' families in the surgical waiting room by a researcher who is pretending to be a relative or friend of a patient in surgery. Usually in these studies permission for the study has been granted by key persons in the institution, such as hospital administration or medical staff, but the actual subjects are unaware of the study. Other such studies have included those where persons have pretended to be patients in order to observe nurse-patient interactions, or have otherwise disguised their true reason for being present in the situation.

The Researcher as the Professional. Studies utilizing participant observation as the data collection method include those where the researcher is normally part of the setting. All attempts to test new nursing interventions without informing patients that they are involved in research fall into this category. Also included are observational studies done by nursing supervisors of their subordinates and data collected by inservice educators of the staff that they are teaching. Data collected by teachers on their students in schools of nursing as well as that collected on practicing nurses have the same basic problem. The subjects do not know that they are research participants because the data collection and sometimes even the experimental intervention is a normal activity for the researcher and thus needs no explanation.

All of these studies share the common denominator of failing to obtain consent from the subjects and thus limiting their right of free choice. In each case, the researcher believes that seeking an informed consent would somehow alter the behavior of the subjects, making the study less meaningful. If this belief can be substantiated, then the proposal can be evaluated for its potential contribution versus the extent to which it imposes on the subjects' time and welfare. The alternatives are either to abandon the research or to carry it out with the subjects' full knowledge and consent.

Coercion of Subjects to Participate

The assumption behind the concept of informed consent is that given sufficient information on which to base a decision, a subjects' consent to participate is free. However, there are various ways in which consent may be partly, or even wholly, coerced by the circumstances under which it is obtained.

Many times the researcher is in a position to require that the subjects participate in the study. For instance, the researcher may be the subject's employer or teacher and thus exert considerable control over the subject. An employer or a teacher may *require* that individuals participate as a condition of remaining an employee or passing a course. Without question, this is coercion.

Another type of coercion occurs when patients are required to give consent to participate in research in order to be accepted as a patient in a particular institution. This might happen in medical centers and specialty hospitals such as those specializing in the treatment of catastrophic illnesses. The patient is likely to feel that his or her "last chance" rests with that institution and therefore feels compelled to consent to anything.

Partial coercion occurs when people are given the option to refuse, but with it the sense that refusal will not go unpunished. For instance, when a nursing supervisor brings questionnaires to a nursing unit, distributes them, and says she will be back to pick them up in an hour, at least some of the nurses are likely to feel that a refusal will offend their supervisor, even though they are given the option, perhaps thinking it will have an effect on their days off or their shift rotation.

Patients are particularly vulnerable to requests to participate in research when the person making the request is someone the patient must depend on for critical needs. The physician and the primary nurse can easily take advantage of a patient's vulnerability.

The ethical issue for the researcher is to recognize that potential subjects are never obligated to assist with research. Many times it will seem obvious that it will be to the advantage of the individual to participate in the research. Perhaps the individual will benefit from extra nursing care or a special teaching program. Perhaps employees will reap the benefits of shorter working hours, less shift rotation, or improved supervision. While all of this may be true, it is still the right of the individuals to decide for themselves; thus, while the advantages of participation can be mentioned as part of the information needed for informed consent, the decision should never be made for the person.

Uninformed Consent

There are cases where consent willingly given to participate in a research project is not *informed* because the subject is not aware of the true nature of the research. There are two methods of obtaining an uninformed consent: one is to give only partial information about the study, usually in general terms; the other is to give false information about the purpose of the study or the procedures that will be followed. Both of these methods of obtaining consent are questionable, in that both inhibit the right of free choice. The use of deception is considered more unethical than the withholding of information, although the line separating the two may be undistinguishable.

Withholding Information. This practice has been widely used in all types of studies where it is believed that complete information about the purpose of the study will influence the subject's response. Thus patients will be told that they will be participating in a study to "improve nursing care," when the actual question could be anything from, "What are patients' attitudes toward male nurses?" to "What is the relationship between ethnic background and perception of pain?"

Another instance of withholding information is found in the use of placebos to compare against the effect of the "real" treatment. It is usual not to inform participants whether they are receiving the placebo or the real treatment. For example, when testing the effect of a new teaching method on diabetic patients' ability to keep their blood sugar under control, patients may not be told whether they are receiving the new or the old teaching method in an attempt to prevent this knowledge from influencing the results. These practices are so widely accepted that the patients' right to complete knowledge before consenting is rarely considered.

Professionals use a number of rationalizations for withholding information from participants. One is that informed consent is only necessary when there is some risk involved for the participant. If the researcher determines that no risk factor exists, they conclude that the subjects do not need complete information about the study.

Another rationalization is that researchers are only obligated to give information that the subject requests about the study, and that the responsibility for informed consent therefore belongs to the subjects. An assumption that often accompanies this thinking is that people are really not interested in the research question, but only in what will happen to them as subjects.

None of these instances give sufficient weight to the right of the individual to make an informed decision. Thus all are questionable practices.

Deceiving the Subject. Not only is information sometimes *withheld* from the subject; *false* information about the study is also given in order to obtain consent. Using deception to gain subject's consent without influencing their behavior might seem far-fetched until you begin to think of some examples of when it might be used. For instance, in a study of mothers' behavior toward their battered children, you might tell the mother that the purpose of the study is to observe the child's behavior, since knowing that she was the subject of the research might not only influence her behavior, but also the likelihood of her giving consent.

A study of the amount of time coronary care nurses spend watching electronic monitors versus interacting with patients might be influenced by the nurses' knowledge of what is being studied. Therefore, a researcher in the CCU might pretend that the study is to collect data on traffic patterns in the Unit at different times of the day.

Studies involving deception of the subjects are frequently addressing controversial issues, such as child-battering, drug abuse, prejudicial or negligent treatment of patients, or in any case where it is assumed that knowledge of the study will cause the subject to adopt a more socially acceptable behavior. Even though the results of these studies can produce far-reaching effects, the practice of deception should be avoided in most cases. In nursing research, diminishing the mutual trust on which patient care is based can rarely, if ever, be justified in terms of the value of the research. Alternatives to deception must be considered and tried.

Stress

Studying the reactions of people to stressful situations is a large subject of nursing research. Rather than being interested in the stress itself, as many social scientists are, nurses are more likely to be interested in methods of assisting people to adapt to stressful situations. In studying patient behaviors, it is not usually necessary for nurse researchers to create stressful situations, since their subjects are under some sort of unusual stress just by being patients. It is necessary, however, to be aware of the possibility of additional stress being created by the research procedures. No research subject should be exposed to physical or emotional stress without his or her informed consent; if the subject is a patient, studies causing additional stress should probably not be conducted at all.

Cases where the study causes stress as a side effect are of concern to nursing research. An example would be an instance where patients was led to believe that their illnesses were not progressing as they should by the nature of the questions that were asked in an interview. These patients may suspect, as a consequence, that they have not been given the whole story by the physician.

Invasion of Privacy

The issue of invasion of privacy has been played up in newspaper headlines and brought into open discussion, particularly regarding offenses by police, credit bureaus, and politicians. It is unlikely that a researcher today would even conceive of using hidden microphones or wiretapping to collect data, although a few years ago these practices were not uncommon. It is generally agreed that everyone has the right to privacy, and that personal information or private affairs are not to be publicly disclosed. Private affairs include such things as personal hygiene, intimate relationships between adults, financial status, religious and political beliefs, and so on. When people are ill, many of their personal affairs become exposed to the health professionals involved in their care. However, it is expected that private affairs of patients remain confidential within the health professions. Therefore, data gathered in the course of one's professional activities may not be used for research without the patient's consent.

Other instances of invasion of privacy may occur when family members or friends are interviewed without the subject's permission; or by observing people in places where they were not expecting it, such as elevators, waiting rooms, or cafeterias. The use of participant observation can provide a special case of invasion of privacy, either when the subjects are unaware that they are being observed, or when they have grown so used to the presence of the observer that their behavior is uninhibited.

Indirect or projective tests of personality or behavior are also a type of invasion of privacy in that they are designed to measure traits that the subjects are unaware of or characteristics that the subjects might wish to conceal. An example of a projective test is the TAT (Thematic Apperception Test), where subjects are asked to tell stories about pictures. Their responses are used to assess the strength of their achievement motivation.

The negative aspects of invasion of privacy come from the ways in which it is used in everyday life, rather than the uses made of data gathered for research. In research, the identity of the individual subject is unimportant; it is the response of one subject in comparison to another or to a group that is of interest to the researcher. When evaluating proposals for which the method of data collection involved some invasion of privacy, it is the researcher's ability to protect the confidentiality of the data that should be evaluated.

Withholding Benefits from Control Subjects

This issue is particularly critical in medical studies where it is apparent that the new treatment would be of value to all the subjects, including the control group. Occasionally a control group is deprived of something they had access to earlier, in order to obtain a more accurate assessment of the new treatment. Both instances provide ethical dilemmas for researchers. However, it must be remembered that the majority of control groups suffer no deprivation.

Sometimes problems with control-group deprivation occur because of the overzealousness of an inexperienced researcher, and, in fact, are not necessary. For example, in a study to test the effectiveness of a pre-operative teaching program on post-operative anxiety, the nursing staff were told not to answer any questions from the patients and families in the control group. This overzealousness deprived the control group of their expected privileges, and in fact, introduced a new variable—deprivation of information—which was not part of the research question. This kind of mistake can easily be picked up in the proposal if the researcher addresses the topic of human rights of all subjects, including the control group.

In some experimental studies, the benefit of the experimental variable is so obvious that those who are cooperating with the researcher in carrying out the study will refuse to deprive the control group of the benefit. This kind of study is particularly difficult for nurses to carry out, since their primary responsibility is the care of patients, and not experimentation. Dedicated nurses would find themselves hard-pressed to deprive a group of patients of an obvious beneficial treatment, such as a simple relaxation exercise that relieves post-operative pain. If this difficulty can be predicted, perhaps control data should be collected prior to introducing the experimental variable, thus avoiding the problem for the nurse.

Sometimes the withholding of benefits from the control group can be rectified at the end of the experiment by making them available at that time. A method of teaching diabetics that proved immensely successful could be provided for the control patients after the data were collected. It should be remembered, however, that this effort must be planned in advance, along with the actual experiment, so that time and money are budgeted for carrying it out.

BALANCING POTENTIAL BENEFIT AGAINST ACTUAL COST

In all disciplines, scientists are obligated to develop new knowledge through research. In any research proposal, the researcher is obligated to weigh the potential contribution of the research, both to the discipline and to society, against the costs to participants in the study. In some cases there is no problem. Full informed consent can be obtained from the participants—they can make a free choice based on sufficient information. In other cases, because of the nature of the question and the procedures necessary to elicit the required data, there is some violation of the rights of the subjects. The benefits of the research must be carefully examined in light of the cost to the subjects.

The Value of the Research Question

The process of weighing the costs and benefits is always a subjective one. The investigator will always be slanted in favor of the research. To reduce subjectivity, three areas should be addressed: *potential contribution to knowledge; practical value to society;* and *benefit to the subject.* The first includes the development of theory to explain nursing practice, and an improvement in the consumer's understanding of health care delivery. The second involves improvement in the delivery of health care to the public, and improved assessment of the health-care needs of ethnic minorities.

The third might be more rapid recovery from illness because of improved nursing care, or increased understanding of preventive health measures. Addressing one or more of these three areas should produce substantial evidence to balance the potential cost to the subject.

The process of balancing potential benefits and costs requires analysis of degree as well as kind of benefit or cost. How important is the problem under study? It is frequently difficult to say. It is expected, however, that questions about *now* issues in nursing will assume more relevance and importance than those that are of interest only to the researcher.

The same question can be asked of the potential cost to the subject. How serious is the potential infringement on the subject's rights? How much harm might it do? Is it likely to be a fleeting inconvenience or a lasting harm?

Answers to both questions will meet with considerable disagreement among colleagues. Once again, it should be emphasized that the researcher is likely to be biased in favor of the research. Therefore, all possible resources should be used to help make the decision to go ahead.

Resources for Decision-Making

Consultation can be obtained from a number of sources to help evaluate the protection of the rights of the subjects in the proposal.

Colleagues. People who are interested in research in the same or similar area are a valuable resource. You may obtain very helpful advice as to how to proceed from other researchers who have faced the same dilemma. There is one shortcoming to using colleagues, and that is that they may be as biased as you are in favor of the proposed research. It is difficult for one who is closely involved in the area to be objective about balancing pluses and minuses, and the tendency might be to weigh the potential contribution as much higher than someone not involved in the area would do.

Consultants. Persons with different backgrounds, from other disciplines, even laymen, can help to assess the importance of both the contribution of the study to society and the potential effect on the subjects. Many nursing studies would benefit from consultation with patients as to their view of the dilemma.

Committees for the Protection of Human Subjects. Medical centers, schools, universities, and many hospitals have formed committees to review research proposals for the purpose of monitoring the protection of subjects' rights. These committees must approve proposals before research can be carried out. They do not relieve the researcher of the responsibility for protecting the rights of the subjects, but they can provide consultation for the researcher. Being accustomed to reviewing proposals, these committees can sometimes help to set the study into proper ethical perspective for the researcher.

There are no easy rules to follow in solving the ethical issues in planning research. The major consideration must always be the safety and well-being of the participants. After this, the research question should be looked at in relation to the rights of the subjects. When there is a conflict, priority must be given to protection of the subjects. When questionable practices are used in lieu of informed consent, they should be such that when informed of them at the end of the study, the subjects find them reasonable and express a willingness to do the same thing again.

MAINTAINING ANONYMITY AND CONFIDENTIALITY

It was mentioned at the beginning of this chapter that the research subject's rights include the right to expect research data to be kept confidential. In addition, the researcher must keep any promise of anonymity made to the subject. These two ideas sound simple, but preserving them may not be so easy.

Plan Ahead.   When promising subjects that they will remain anonymous and the data will be confidential, it is wise to have planned in advance for the possible problems that might arise to prevent you from keeping these promises. For instance, the institution where you plan to collect the data may expect you to share it with their administration. Parents may expect to have access to research data involving their children. Other researchers may request your data to use in their own research. None of these possibilities needs to be a problem if you have planned ahead. The institution must understand and agree that they will have access only to the summarized results and not to the raw data. If this is not acceptable, then do not promise anonymity to the subjects, or select another institution. Whatever the request for access to the data might be, however innocuous, no information should be released without the subject's permission.

Data Banks.   A data bank is any collection of coded information about individuals kept in a form that is easily retrievable. Computers make the formulation of data banks an easy task. The potential value of data banks to research is enormous. At present, most data banks in existence belong to various government agencies, such as the Internal Revenue Service. The compilation of data banks by survey researchers is just in the beginning stages.

It is possible, however, that a data bank might request you to contribute data from your study for the use of other researchers. Until methods are perfected for coding and protecting the identity of the subjects, however, it would be wise to avoid contributing to data banks. At least do not do so without making sure that your subjects' identities are protected.

Legal Problems. All researchers should be aware of the fact that the confidentiality of research data is not recognized by law. This means that research data can be subpoenaed for use in court, and that a researcher may be required to testify about people who have been research subjects. When your subjects are heroin addicts, child abusers, and others who may have broken the law, you need to consider the possibility that you may be required to surrender your records or testify against your subjects.

Publication. Before they consent to participate, your subjects need to be made aware that you intend to publish the results of your study. In studies of groups of people, it is frequently impossible to maintain anonymity of the group when publishing your findings. It may be the only group of its kind, so that even with disguising the names and location, it is possible to identify the members. This can prove embarrassing to the individual members, and they need to be aware of the possibility before they consent to be studied.

Your method of data analysis can cause loss of anonymity for your subjects if you are not careful. If, for instance, you are reporting findings in an attitude study of staff nurses, and you cross-tabulate them by shift, unit, and position, you may run into the possibility that there is only one R.N. on the night shift on a particular unit, and her responses will be easily identified. You may find that in order to maintain confidentiality, you will have to omit some of your data analysis from the published report.

All of these potential difficulties in maintaining confidentiality can be avoided by planning ahead. In this case it is not enough just to "not promise what you can't deliver." The onus is on the researcher to inform the subject that some or all of the data will become public knowledge, or that some individuals other than the researcher will have access to it. Otherwise, the subject has the right to assume that all data will be kept confidential.

RECOMMENDED READING

American Nurses Association. *The Nurse in Research: ANA Guidelines on Ethical Values,* 1968.

Creighton, Helen, and Armington, Catherine. "Legal Concerns of Research and Nurse Researchers." *Issues in Research: Social, Professional, and Methodological.* Selected Papers from the ANA Council of Nurse Researchers Program Meeting, August 22–24, 1973, pp. 18–30.

Fleming, Juanita. "Human Rights and Ethical Concerns of Scientists." *Issues in Research: Social Professional and Methodological.* Selected Papers from the ANA Council of Nurse Researchers Program Meeting, August 22–24, 1973, pp. 36–49.

U.S. Department of Health, Education and Welfare. *The Institutional Guide to DHEW Policy on Protection of Human Subjects.* Washington, D.C.: Government Printing Office, 1971.

XIV.

Planning for Analysis of Data

Inferential Analysis
1. Testing Hypotheses
   a. The Null Hypothesis
   b. Parametric and Nonparametric Statistical Tests

2. Choosing a Statistical Test: What Does Your Hypothesis Ask?
   a. Difference between Two Groups
   b. Difference among Multiple Groups
   c. Correlation between Variables
   d. Estimation of Population Parameters from Sample Data

3. Be Sure You Can Answer Your Question

The Answer Is in the Question
1. Level I Questions
2. Level II Questions
3. Level III Questions

The goal of analysis is to summarize the data so that they provide answers to the research question. Your plan for data analysis is derived from your question, your design, your method of data collection and the level of measurement of your data. All previous choices that you have made in these areas will direct and limit your choice of data analysis techniques.

The basic differentiation in plans for analysis is between *descriptive* and *inferential* analysis. Descriptive analysis provides description of the data *from your particular sample,* and therefore your conclusions must refer only to your sample. Inferential analysis, on the other hand, provides statistical support for the answer to your research question, allowing you to draw inferences about the larger population from your sample data.

Descriptive analysis includes content analysis of unstructured data, which results in a summarization of the data into categories. It also includes presenting categories of data in tables or graphs that provide a pictorial description of the sample; the use of descriptive statistics to further describe individual variables; and the use of statistical analysis for the purpose of looking for relationships among categories or variables.

Inferential analysis always involves the use of statistical tests, either to test for significant relationships among variables or to find statistical support for the hypotheses. In either case, your purpose is to support your explanation of the relationships among your variables, thus testing the conceptual or theoretical framework behind your study.

The data analysis is intended to provide the answer to your research question. Thus it must be planned ahead along with the rest of your study. Too often, researchers stop planning after they complete their plans for data collection, thinking that the analysis can be done later. "Later" may bring a rude awakening when they suddenly discover that the data collected will not provide the answers needed. Then it is too late to plan the analysis. Keep in mind that you want to answer your question. Critically examine your data analysis plan with this thought in mind, and you will not become bogged down in a mass of irrelevant statistics.

This chapter will present descriptive analysis first, followed by a discussion of inferential analysis. Since there are many excellent references for the actual performance of statistical tests, the tests will be discussed here only as they relate to answering the research question, and then only in general terms.

DESCRIPTIVE ANALYSIS

Within descriptive analysis there is a wide range of choices for planning the analysis of the data, from simple to complex. But descriptive methods all have one thing in common—they summarize the data. The types of summarization range from using content analysis to organize the data into categories to the use of descriptive statistics such as frequency distributions and measures of central tendency. A descriptive analysis might also include looking for statistical relationships among categories or variables.

The type of analysis you choose depends on how precisely you were able to measure your variables. Very imprecise, crude measurement is apt to be nonquantifiable, or quantifiable only at the nominal level. Therefore, the analysis is limited to depicting the data summary in charts or graphs. You can categorize, list, and describe your findings, giving a graphic representation of how your sample might fall in each category. Then all that is left for you to do when you have collected your data is describe how each case was different from or similar to each other case and on what dimension.

For some studies, this analysis technique is sufficient. Particularly if you are using a new or different way of categorizing and describing your variable, or if you are describing something for the first time. On the other hand, you might want to plan to look for which categories are most frequently associated with others, which always stand alone, and which seem to vary depending upon the interaction of one or more factors. Since you are exploring relationships, all possible permutations of these relationships need to be described and given some kind of rationale. Exploratory studies require the most time-consuming and detailed analysis of data of any type of research. Do not be fooled by the simplicity of the design; the analysis is the hardest part of this type of study, simply because you know so little about what you are studying. And obviously, from the literature review, neither does anyone else. Therefore, it is up to you, the one who asked the question, to describe in detail everything you observed so that your study is informative and capable of being replicated.

The time and effort involved in the analysis of exploratory studies cannot be overemphasized. The simplicity and flexibility of the design lead many novice researchers to think that exploratory studies are the easiest to conduct. These people have obviously not considered the analysis of data. Take, for instance, an exploratory study of stress reactions of hospitalized children. This study can be likened to a series of in-depth case studies of individuals undergoing the stress of hospitalization. Initially, the subjects are chosen for their similarity to one another: they are all children, and all are hospitalized patients. Perhaps they even have similar diagnoses. However, as soon as you begin to observe them in depth, differences begin to emerge. The more you observe, the more differences you will see. When you have finished data collection, there will be a tremendous volume of material describing a lot of different children and their reactions to a stressful situation. These data could be reported as a series of case studies in story form with no analysis on your part. But as an exploratory researcher, you are obligated to organize the data from these individual children in such a way that the similarities and trends can be examined as well as any differences. Further, when differences are described, they must be looked at in terms of other descriptive characteristics of the children so that tentative hypotheses can be formulated for further study.

In descriptive analysis, the process is very similar in all types of studies, but more precise measurement enables you to use more techniques in your analysis. The choice always depends first on your question, and then the type of measurement you plan to use.

Getting the Overall Picture

In any type of study, plan to spend some time just looking at your data. With unstructured data, reading through all your material will give you ideas for categories and themes. With structured data you will also get a general impression of the material that will help you sort out what to do first. Take this opportunity, also, to look for gaps in the data. Are there any unanswered questions in your questionnaire? Is there a missing sequence in your field notes? Now is the time to supply the missing items. If this is not possible, then those subjects for which data are missing may have to be dropped from the analysis, or at least analyzed separately.

Unstructured Data: Content Analysis

In exploratory descriptive studies, and also in many descriptive surveys, the data are unstructured and not immediately subject to summarization. The verbatim recording of conversations or reports of observations do not, in themselves, provide the answer to the research question. First they must be categorized, summarized, and tabulated using a process called *content analysis*. This extremely demanding process is probably the most difficult technique of data analysis, and is one in which the researcher plays a highly creative role. Theory is sometimes developed on the basis of content analysis of unstructured data, frequently resulting in concepts and operational definitions.

If the study has a conceptual or theoretical framework, the researcher can set up classifications or categories in advance, simplifying, somewhat, the process of content analysis. The researcher will plan to go through the data to see if the observations fit into the categories and with what frequency. For example, using the nursing process as a conceptual framework within which to analyze nurses' notes, four categories might be derived: 1) assessment; 2) diagnosis; 3) intervention; and 4) evaluation. The data for this study would be nurses' notes. The content analysis would involve taking each statement made by the nurse in the notes and deciding to which of the four categories it belongs. This requires that precise definitions for each of the four categories be developed in the research plan. Without clear definitions, a statement such as "Incision appears to be healing" might be assessment or evaluation.

When planning to do content analysis, you must first decide which aspect of the content you are interested in classifying. The content can be divided into two broad categories: (1) the actual semantic content of the subjects' responses and (2) the feeling or attitude being conveyed by the subjects' responses. In some studies these categories may be combined. Let's examine each in turn.

Semantic Content.   In content analysis, you will be interested most often in analyzing the statements made by your subjects. Take, for example, the following responses to the question asked of hospitalized patients, "What kinds of nurses work on this floor?"

a. They're O.K.
b. Mostly blacks, maybe a few Chicanos.
c. None of 'em know what they're doing most of the time.
d. I could say a lot about the nurses around here, but I don't want to cause any trouble.
e. They're very nice, especially at night.
f. Blacks and Mexicans, and maybe a few whites.
g. I don't know, I'm new here.
h. Very pretty ones.

When you asked this question, you obviously were not seeking factual information about the nurses, but rather looking for what patients thought was important. If your data contain several hundred responses such as these, it is easy to see that in order to answer the research question, you must put them into a limited number of categories suggested by the question itself.

If your question was, "What awareness do patients have of a nurses' appearance?", the categories to start with are: 1) mentions appearance and 2) does not mention appearance. These are simple categories into which every response can be classified; the results will tell you how important a nurses' appearance seems to be in relation to all other qualities a patient will mention. Notice that these categories have the same theme: both relate to the mention of appearance. This is an important criteria for a set of categories—it must measure a single dimension or theme. A set of categories is a nominal scale, after all, and therefore must classify according to a single theme, and have no overlap between categories. The same scale cannot measure appearance and ethnic group. These are different concepts, and each requires its own set of categories.

Using the same patient responses, let's assume that the research question was a more exploratory one: "What are patients' impressions of nurses?" Here the job of classifying the responses into semantic categories becomes more complex. The first step is to scan the responses to get a feel for the various kinds of statements made by the patients. You might notice several statements referring to the nurses' ethnic backgrounds. A set of categories could be developed to cover this theme. For instance:

a. mentions ethnic background of nurses
b. does not mention ethnic background

If these two categories do not provide enough information about the patients' responses, more detailed subcategories can be developed, such as:

a. mentions blacks, but no other groups
b. mentions blacks and Chicanos, but no other groups
c. mentions groups other than blacks or Chicanos
d. mentions blacks, Chicanos, and other group(s)
e. does not mention ethnic background

These categories form a set into which all the responses can be classified, and they measure a single theme—ethnic response.

Since the question asked for the patients' general impressions about nurses, further analysis of the content is necessary. Other themes will appear as you scan the data. For instance, you might find that some patients mentioned the knowledge or skill of the nurses. A set of categories could be developed to cover this area. Another theme might be the nurses' manner, as indicated by descriptions such as *warm, cold, hurried, patient,* etc. You also might want to look at reasons for not responding to the question, for which you could develop categories like:

a. responded to question
b. did not respond, no reason given

    c. did not respond, said, "I don't know"
    d. did not respond, indicated he/she did know but did not want
       to be involved
    e. did not respond, other reason given

This process must be continued until all possible themes have been exhausted. For exploratory studies with masses of unstructured data, the process is complex, difficult and extremely time-consuming.

Feeling Tone.   Analysis for feeling tone is used to describe the attitude or feeling conveyed by the response or behavior being analyzed. Frequently it is done in conjunction with the semantic content analysis, so that both the content and the feeling conveyed by that content are looked at together. Or it may be that the research question only asks about feeling tone.

    When looking for feeling tone, the first step must be to decide on the *unit of content* to be analyzed: the entire response or individual words and phrases that make up the response. This decision depends on whether you want a general impression or a specific one.

    The next step is to decide on the categories to be used. A set of categories must be developed into which all the responses will fit. For example, you might want to use positive and negative or passive and aggressive feeling tone as the theme for your categories. To illustrate the process, let's use some patients' responses to the question, "What did you think of the services you received at the family planning clinic?"

    a. I thought it was great, but didn't understand it all.
    b. The nurses were nice, they were really interested in my
       problem.
    c. Now I really understand contraception.
    d. The classes were really good. I liked all the lectures, but I sure
       wish they'd learn how to make good coffee. It was terrible.
    e. There were five classes and each one had its own topic. Each
       person then saw the doctor and the nurse.
    f. It was a total waste of time.

The unit of content for analysis of these responses will be the entire statement. The first two categories that come to mind are *positive* and *negative*. Reading through the responses, however, it quickly becomes apparent that some responses, such as *a* and *d*, are partly negative and partly positive; therefore, an intermediate category is needed for "mixed" responses. These three categories are sufficient until you reach *e*. This response does not seem to fit; in fact, it is devoid of any feeling at all. A new category must be developed for this response. It might be called *neutral* and be defined as "a response unrelated to the theme being analyzed." Now the set of categories looks like this:

1. positive: a response with only favorable perceptions of the clinic sessions
2. mixed: a response containing both positive and negative perceptions
3. negative: a response giving only negative feelings about the clinic
9. neutral: a response which lacks indication of the theme being analyzed.

(Notice that the neutral category is given the number "9" so that it is apparent that it falls outside the categories based on the positive-negative theme.)

Now the sample responses can be classified quite easily into the four categories:

a. I thought it was great, but didn't understand it all. *Mixed* (2)
b. The nurses were nice, they were really interested in my problem. *Positive* (1)
c. Now I really understand contraception. *Positive* (1)
d. The classes were really good. I liked all the lectures, but I sure wish they'd learn how to make good coffee. It was terrible. *Mixed* (2)
e. There were five classes and each one had its own topic. Each person then saw the doctor and the nurse. *Neutral* (9)
f. It was a total waste of time. *Negative* (3)

In this example, changing the unit of content to individual phrases eliminates the need for the *mixed* category. Each phrase would then be looked at individually and classified so that response *a* then forms two phrases. The first phrase, "I thought it was great," is then classified as *positive*. The second phrase, "Didn't understand it all," becomes *negative*. This approach will allow some weighting of the responses, in that each is given a score. Thus several positive statements and one negative statement will be weighted toward the positive end of the continuum. This is a factor to consider when choosing the best unit of content.

Coding. The actual procedure of categorizing data is called *coding*.

Through this process the raw data are put into categories that have symbols, usually numbers, enabling the frequencies within the categories to be counted.

The coding process requires judgment on the part of the coder. A decision must be made on every response as to which category it belongs. So that the decision can be as objective as possible, the definitions of the categories must be complete and unambiguous. Since definitions must apply to the immediate data, examples are needed from the data that represent typical responses for that category. For example, the category *mentions manner of nurse* might be defined as "any mention of the quality of the nurse's manner toward patients, such as being too busy to answer questions; kind and gentle; cold and unfeeling; warm and friendly."

Special problems arise with respect to the reliability of coding of unstructured data, mostly from the subjective nature of the coding process. These problems can appear in many forms. First of all, the recording of the raw data may be inadequate. Perhaps the observations are incomplete or illegible. Perhaps key words are missing that would have clarified the data for the coder. This can be avoided by frequent editing of the data during the collection. If you are recording observations, have someone else read your recordings frequently and describe them in their own words. This will give you a good idea of whether your description is adequately conveying the behavior that you observed.

Another major area of difficulty comes from the definition of the categories. Are they sufficiently detailed and do they make sense to the coder? Do the categories represent the theme that they are describing, and are they relevant to the purpose of the research? These questions can only be answered by the investigator.

The training of coders is extremely important. After the categories are explained, the coders then need a chance to practice on a sample of the data. Problems that arise should be discussed in a group to ensure that all coders receive the same information. The results of the practice coding are compared, and practice continues until inconsistencies have been eliminated. When the actual process of coding the data begins, periodic checks for consistency should be made to ensure the continued reliability of the coding.

The simplest measure of reliability of coded data is obtained by calculating the percentage of agreement between two or more coders rating the same data. This check on the consistency of coding is required for all content analysis, whether several coders are used or the researcher does all coding personally. If you plan to code your own data, you must also plan to have a random sample of the data analyzed by one or more other people, using a procedure similar to *equivalency* in estimating the reliability of instruments. Keep in mind that your assistant coders will need training and practice in order to do a good job.

Validity in Content Analysis.   This refers to the extent to which the categories represent the theme or concept upon which they are based. In studies where the categories are based on a theoretical or conceptual framework, their content validity must be established. This is done by explaining where they came from and why they fit the theory or concept. In addition, it must be shown that they are measuring a single theme or concept. If, for instance, you are classifying nurses' responses to physicians as *assertive, passive,* and *aggressive,* you must first relate the three categories to your conceptual framework and, second, show that they are a continuum measuring one dimension of the theme and not three independent concepts.

In exploratory studies that do not have conceptual frameworks, face validity for the categories must be demonstrated. This is done by developing a rationale for the categories and their definitions, and showing that they are appropriate to the data. Face validity is further supported by the ease with which the responses can be classified into the categories, and the apparent relevance of the categories to the research question.

Structured Data: Statistical Analysis

Cross-tabulation.   The old saying that a "picture is worth a thousand words" describes the reason for developing tables. A cross-tabulation is simply a tabular presentation of data, either in frequency or percentage form or both, in which variables can be examined for any relationships among them. Cross-tabulations enable the researcher to not only look at the relations among variables, but also to organize the data into a convenient form for statistical analysis.

The variables used to cross-tabulate the data are either the categories resulting from content analysis or the variables found in the purpose of the study. Although cross-tabulations are mainly used with nominal data, they can also be used as a first step in more complex analysis.

Imagine a descriptive study of stress in which the purpose is to describe patients' reactions to stress while in the dental chair. Data will be collected by observing nonverbal behavior, and measuring blood pressure, pulse, and palmar sweat volume. Data will be compiled on the type of procedures and instruments used by the dentist, the length of the procedures, and demographic variables from the patients. In this descriptive study, you know in advance what you will observe and how, and what instruments will be used to collect data. Most of the data will be in numerical form. In developing a plan to analyze the data from this study, you would start by cross-tabulating the variables.

The simplest cross-tabulation is a 2 × 2 table. In the dental patient study, let's look at nonverbal behavior (relaxed or tense) according to whether or not the dentist used an anesthetic.

Table 1

Frequencies of Nonverbal Indicators of Stress with Use/Nonuse of Local Anesthetic

	ANESTHETIC	NO ANESTHETIC	TOTAL
Relaxed	47	35	82
Tense	5	21	26
Total	52	56	108

In this example, the categories are set up using variables found in the purpose of the study. In another study, they could just as easily be the categories that resulted from content analysis. The categories used in cross-tabulation must meet the same criteria as those developed in content analysis: they must be independent, mutually exclusive, and constructed so that there is a category for all observations. (In Table 1, there is no category for general anesthetic, so it is possible that it does not meet all the criteria.)

Cross-tabulations can be used to describe three or four variables, each one of which has multiple categories. Theoretically, it is possible to cross-tabulate any number of variables, but when more than three are used, the table becomes confusing to read and therefore loses its major value, which is to simplify the data.

Table 2 illustrates the cross-tabulation of three variables. In this case, increase in apical pulse is used as a measure of patient stress during dental work, and is examined in relation to the age and sex of the patients.

Table 2

Relationships among Age, Sex, and Average Increase in Apical Pulse during Dental Work

	MALES			FEMALES		
	20–30	31–40	41–50	20–30	31–40	41–50
Apical Pulse Increase >10/min.	25	60	10	30	40	25
<10/min.	75	40	90	70	60	75

It is now possible to compare males and females in each of the age groups on apical pulse increase. This can be done for any number of sets of variables that you wish to examine. The tabulation can be done entirely by hand or by a computer. Hand tabulation has the advantage of completely familiarizing you with your data. The usefulness of many combinations of variables can be seen more easily when you hand tabulate the data. Using a computer is much faster, of course, particularly when a canned program for cross-tabulation is available, but selection and screening of variables to be tabulated must be done in advance; the machine will not do it for you.

If cross-tabulation is appropriate to your study, *it must be planned in advance.* As we pointed out in the discussion on sample size, the number of variables you plan to cross-tabulate can affect your sample size. Therefore, it wise to plot out your tables ahead of time. Make up some fictitious data while you are planning your tables. This will give you a good idea of what your results will look like, and you can then be sure that they will provide the answer to your research question.

Descriptive Statistics. The various methods of summarizing numerical data for descriptive purposes will be briefly discussed here, since they can readily be found in any statistics text.

Measures of central tendency—mean, median, and mode—isolate one response that is representative of the sample. Each requires a specific level of measurement. To have a meaningful measure of central tendency, the appropriate one must be used. The mean requires interval or ratio data; the median, ordinal data; and the mode, nominal data.

To arrive at a mean, the scores of the sample are totaled and the sum is divided by the number of scores. It represents the "average" score of the sample. You can use the mean with physiological variables such as blood pressure, pulse, and blood volume, or with age, income, time, and other interval data.

The median is meant to be used with ordinal data, although you can certainly use it with interval and ratio data as well. The median is simply a point on a scale where half of the scores fall above and half fall below. You can use the median with any rating scale.

When the measurement scale is nominal, the mode is the only appropriate measure of central tendency. The mode indicates the category that occurs with greatest frequency. In Table 1 (p. 152), the categories of *anesthetic* and *no anesthetic* were nominal data. The measure of central tendency from the data in that table indicates that *no anesthetic* is the modal category, since the majority of subjects fall in that category.

Measures of variation describe how widely the individuals in the sample vary. Are your subjects quite similar to one another or is there a great diversity among them? The most often-used measures of variation are the *range,* the *quartile range,* and the *standard deviation.*

The range shows the highest and lowest scores in the group, or the extremes of variation. The range can be used with ordinal, interval, or ratio data. As an example, you might say, "The ages of the subjects ranged from 3 months to 97 years." As you can see, the range is affected by extreme cases, and gives no indication of what lies between the highest and lowest scores.

The quartile range gives the middle points between which half of the subjects fall. For instance, if the ages of subjects range from 3 months to 97 years, the quartile range might be from 45 to 60 years. That tells you that one fourth of the sample is below 45, one fourth is above 60, and the remaining half is between 45 and 60. Now you have a much better picture of the age range than you did before.

The standard deviation, on the other hand, is a measure of the average distance of each subject from the group mean. Like the mean, the standard deviation requires interval or ratio data. The standard deviation derives from the normal curve, so you know that approximately 75% of the sample falls within two standard deviations above or below the mean. Thus, if the mean age is 52 years, and the standard deviation is 4 years, you know that 75% of the sample is between 44 and 60 years of age (8 years, or two standard deviations, above and below the mean age of 52).

If you have nominal data, the number of categories needed to represent a theme or concept indicates how much variation there is in the sample. If two diagnostic categories are sufficient to represent the range of diagnoses in the sample, that indicates less variation in diagnosis than if several are required.

Looking for Relationships.   In descriptive studies, the plan is to describe the variables and also to look for significant relationships among them. For instance, you may wish to know if patients' ethnic backgrounds are related to their responses to group therapy. Or you might wonder if education and income level are associated with career choice in high school students. You might have a long list of demographic variables, and you want to know if any one or a combination of these variables are related to a student's success in nursing school.

There are several statistical methods of showing the relationships between variables, and some of the more commonly-used ones will be discussed. Remember, however, that in descriptive studies, no attempt is made to draw conclusions about causal relationships from the data. Rather, hypotheses are formulated from statistically significant relationships, and these relationships are later tested in more controlled studies from which causal relationships might be developed.

   Chi-square analysis is designed for analyzing categories of nominal data that have been set up in cross-tabulation form. The Chi-square test is based on the assumption that if there is no relationship between two or more variables, then the likelihood of the individuals in your sample falling into the various categories of each variable is a chance occurrence. For example, in Table 3, if there is no relationship between stress (as measured by relaxed or tense) and use of local anesthetic, then the 52 subjects who received local anesthetic should have an equal chance of falling into either category of stress; *this chance would be the same for the No Anesthetic group.* The Chi-square test picks up the significance of any true departures from the frequencies that would be expected by chance. When you find significantly more subjects in one category than would be expected by chance, you can interpret this finding as an association between the two variables being tested.

Table 3
Frequencies of Nonverbal Indicators of Stress and Use
of Local Anesthetic

	ANESTHETIC	NO ANESTHETIC	TOTAL
Relaxed	47	35	82
Tense	5	21	26
Total	52	56	108
Chi-square = 11.5, d.f. = 1, p = .01			

   In Table 3, a Chi-square analysis has been done using the method described by Seigel.* The results indicate that there is a significant relationship between local anesthetic and nonverbal indicators of stress. The probability of the sample falling into the categories of *relaxed* and *tense* as they would simply by chance was less than .05 (the actual probability was .01), and therefore is considered to be statistically significant.

   If your data consist of pairs of numbers, that is, two variables have been measured for each subject in your sample, then a *measure of correlation* can be used to tell you if these two variables are related to each other. For example, you might be planning to measure IQ and attitude toward women's rights; or blood pressure and temperature; or self-image and body weight. A correlational test will tell you whether these pairs of variables have a tendency to *vary together*—does blood pressure increase (or decrease) as the body temperature goes up; is a negative self-image related to being overweight (does self-image go down as weight goes up)? If the direction of the relationship is *positive,*

---

*Seigel, Sidney, *Nonparametric Statistics for the Behavioral Sciences,* (New York: McGraw Hill, 1956), pp. 104–110.

(both variables increase or decrease together), the numerical value of the correlation will be positive (somewhere between 0 and +1). If the direction of the relationship is *negative* (as one variable increases the other decreases), the correlation will be negative (somewhere between 0 and −1). The strength of the relationship between the two variables is greater as the correlation approaches +1 or =1, so that a correlation of .9 is much stronger than a correlation of .3.

All measures of correlation require at least ordinal data. If your planned data will be in nominal categories, use Chi-square. If you plan ordinal data, you must have at least seven points on your scale so that there will be enough variation in the scores from your sample for you to see if the two variables are varying in the same direction. If you have only three points on your scale (such as high, medium and low), there will not be enough variation in your sample to be able to use correlation. Once again, go back to Chi-square.

The appropriate correlation test to use with interval or ratio data is the *Pearson r.* This test requires that the data from *both variables* be on at least an interval scale, and that the data be normally distributed.

If one or both of your variables are to be measured on an ordinal scale, one of the nonparametric tests of correlation must be used (see pages 158–159 for explanation of parametric and nonparametric tests). The *Spearmen rank correlation* is the one most often used. This test is 91% as efficient as the *Pearson r,* which makes it a powerful nonparametric test. To use the Spearmen rank correlation, you will have to rank your subjects on both variables according to how they scored on your ordinal scale. The test then substitutes the ranks for the actual scores, thus solving the problem created by the unequal distances between the points on an ordinal scale.

INFERENTIAL ANALYSIS

In explanatory studies, it is not enough just to describe the data; you must also draw conclusions from that data. Statistical inference, which is based on probability theory, is the process of generalizing from sample observations to whole populations. The tools of statistics help to identify valid generalizations, and those that are likely to stand up under further study.

A researcher plans an experiment. Each research subject is seated in a room with two doors, one blue and one yellow. For ten minutes, loud music is played over the intercom. Then a voice tells the subject to leave the room. The researcher notes which door each subject chooses. When this experiment was done with ten subjects, seven subjects chose the blue door. The researcher concluded that the loud music causes people to choose a blue door over a yellow one. Is this a valid generalization? Of course not. The fact is that those results could be purely chance happenings.

Now consider another experiment: a drug was injected into ten healthy subjects. Within five minutes, seven were vomiting and the other three were apparently fine. The researcher concluded that the drug causes vomiting. Recalling the previous experiment with the blue and yellow doors, would you argue that the results of this experiment could also easily have occurred by chance? Why or why not? Let's examine the probabilities.

In the first experiment each person had a fifty-fifty chance of choosing the blue door *without the music*. Seven out of ten is not enough to show a relationship between music and the color of the door when five of the ten are expected to choose either door by chance. In the drug experiment, however, the chance that seven out of ten persons would have started to vomit *without exposure to the drug* are extremely slim, perhaps one in a thousand. Therefore, seven out of ten in this case may be conclusive evidence that the vomiting was caused by the drug. The results of these two experiments must be measured against different probabilities. Statistical analysis provides the means of eliminating most of the subjectivity that goes into the researcher's conclusions, thus separating science from opinion. This is done by using statistical models against which the results of research can be compared.

Because statistical procedures dictate some of the conditions for collecting the evidence, they must be part of the research plan. If planning data analysis is left until after the data are collected, it often happens that the optimal statistical technique cannot be used because some necessary condition of data collection was overlooked.

Testing of Hypotheses

The overall aim of explanatory research is to determine the *acceptability* of hypotheses. The outcome of the study may be to retain, revise, or reject the hypothesis and the theory from which it was derived. To reach an objective conclusion, there must be an objective procedure for either rejecting or accepting that hypothesis. This procedure is based on the data to be collected, and on the amount of risk the researcher is willing to take that the decision to accept or reject the hypothesis will not be correct.

The Null Hypothesis. The first step in planning a decision-making statistical procedure is to state the *null hypothesis*. Null hypotheses always state the opposite of what you expect to find, which usually means stating that there will be no relationship between variables. The reason for using null hypotheses is that statistical tests are designed to reject rather than accept hypotheses. In this sense, rejection is an action word, whereas acceptance is passive. Active rejection of the null hypothesis is as close as you can come to "proving" your hypothesis. You never actively reject your research hypothesis, since it is never directly tested; only the null hypothesis is directly tested. Your goal in statistical analysis is to reject the null hypothesis, thus giving support to your research hypothesis as the alternative. Failing to reject the null hypothesis means only that you failed to support your research hypothesis with this particular study, and leaves the door open for you to test it again under other circumstances.

If your hypothesis states, "During dental procedures, those patients given a local anesthetic will exhibit less stress than those not given a local anesthetic," the null hypothesis would be written as: "There will be no difference in stress exhibited by patients receiving local anesthetic and those not receiving local anesthetic during dental procedures." There are two possible alternatives to this null hypothesis:

(1) Patients given a local anesthetic will exhibit *more* stress than those not given a local anesthetic; and
(2) Patients given a local anesthetic will exhibit *less* stress than those not given a local anesthetic.

Since this latter alternative is the one predicted by your research hypothesis, you will apply a "one-tailed test," which will reject the null hypothesis only if there is less stress among the local anesthetic group.

Two types of error can be made when testing the null hypothesis. The first, called *Type I error,* is to reject the null hypothesis when it is actually true. The *level of significance* that you select for your statistical analysis is the probability that Type I error might occur. If the level of significance is .05, the researcher runs the risk that five times out of a hundred the null hypothesis might be rejected when it is actually true. You always determine the level of significance in advance so that the decision to reject or accept the null hypothesis remains objective.

The second type of error (*Type II error*) is to accept the null hypothesis when it is actually false and should have been rejected. The probability of committing a Type II error can be decreased by increasing the sample size, which is another reason for having as large a sample as possible.

Parametric and Nonparametric Statistical Tests.   Every statistical test is based on certain assumptions that tell under what conditions the test is valid. The line between parametric and nonparametric statistics is fuzzy, but it is generally agreed that parametric tests are based on strong assumptions about the population from which the observations (measurements of the variable) were drawn. If the population meets these assumptions, the parametric test is very powerful, and hence the most likely one to reject a null hypothesis when it is in fact false. Nonparametric tests are based on fewer assumptions and are therefore less powerful. They can, however, be used to analyze data from populations about which very little is known. Since the nonparametric test is less powerful, it is safer to use with data from unknown populations because the risk of error will be less.

The parametric test can be used if the population meets the following assumptions of parametric statistics:

(1) *Known Distribution:* The distribution of the variable in the population is known. For many tests, the variable must be normally distributed in the population. The sample then must be randomly selected so that the sample distribution is the same as that for the population.

(2) *Equal Variances:* When two or more groups are being compared on some variable, it is assumed that the variances of scores for the variable are the same among the groups. In other words, the variances are homogeneous from group to group.

(3) *Equal Intervals:* Because of the arithmetic operations used in computing parametric tests, the variables must be measured on an interval or ratio scale.

These assumptions are not actually tested during data analysis, but rather are assumed to be true or present in the situation. Therefore, the results of a parametric tests have to be interpreted according to whether your data meet the assumptions of the test. If it does not, your results may be in error.

Nonparametric tests do not specify conditions about the parameters of the population from which the sample was drawn. They are sometimes said to be "distribution-free," and thus can be used when you do not know the distribution of the population. Also, there are nonparametric tests for use with nominal and ordinal data. In behavioral research, it is frequently difficult to achieve a level of measurement that permits the use of parametric tests. Therefore, nonparametric tests assume a prominent role in data analysis.

Choosing a Statistical Test: What Does Your Hypothesis Ask?

Although the field of statistical analysis is quite complex, the beginning researcher can use some simple guidelines to look for appropriate techniques to use. The best indication of what general technique to use can be found in your own hypothesis. Look at what it says. Are you looking for a significant difference between *two groups* or *several* groups? Are you interested in *significant correlations* between (or among) variables? Or are you trying to *estimate* what the population is like from findings in your sample? The technique you choose will depend on which of these questions your hypothesis is asking. Let's look at each one individually.

Difference Between Two Groups.   In some studies the subjects are randomly assigned to two groups, one of which is subjected to an experimental independent variable. In other studies, the sample is selected from two populations, for example, two ethnic groups or two educational groups. Both types of studies are interested in the same kind of data analysis. They ask, "Is there a difference between the two groups?"

The *t* test is the classic technique for analyzing the differences between the means of two groups. It is a powerful parametric test, and thus the data must meet the three assumptions listed earlier (the scores are from normally distributed populations with equal variances, measured on an interval scale).

If your data do not meet these assumptions, a nonparametric test such as the *Fisher exact probability* test or the *Mann-Whitney U* test can be used to test for a significant difference between the two groups.

Sometimes you have two sets of scores from the same group, such as "before-and-after" measurements of some variable. In this case, you are looking for a change in scores from one measurement time to another, and you want to know if the change is statistically significant. Often a *difference score* will be obtained for each subject by subtracting one measurement from the other. The *t* test can be used to test for the significance of the difference if the assumptions are met. When the *t* test cannot be used, nonparametric tests for ordinal data include the sign test and the *Wilcoxin* test. The *McNemar chi-square* test can be used with nominal data. These tests are all designed to analyze the significance of the difference in two sets of scores from the same group of subjects.

Difference Among Multiple Groups.   The hypothesis of your study may be directed at whether several independent groups should be regarded as coming from the same population (in relation to the variable being studied), or whether the differences between them indicate that they represent different populations. For instance, your hypothesis might predict that patients from different ethnic groups will select different health care systems.

The usual parametric test for deciding whether several groups have come from the same population is the one-way analysis of variance, or F test. The usual assumptions for parametric tests are required for analysis of variance. If these do not hold, there are several nonparametric tests from which to choose. For nominal data, the chi-square test can be used with multiple groups. Table 4 gives an example of what the chi-square table might look like.

Table 4
Frequency of Selecting a Private Physician, Government System, or Health Maintenance Organization by Subjects from Five Ethnic Groups

HEALTH CARE SYSTEM	WASP	ASIAN	BLACK	AMER- IND.	LATINO	TOTAL
Private Physician	14	12	10	2	6	44
Government System	1	2	11	25	4	43
Health Maint. Organization	3	14	20	20	1	58
Total	18	28	41	47	11	145

The Chi-square test tells you whether ethnic groups choose any of the health care systems more often than would be expected by chance.

If the data are on ordinal scales, the *Kruskal-Wallis one-way analysis of variance by ranks* can be used. This technique tests the null hypothesis that the groups come from the same population, or from identical populations with respect to the variable being measured. It is the most powerful of the nonparametric tests for independent groups.

Correlation Between Variables. Establishing that a correlation exists between two variables may be the purpose of your study, and your hypothesis predicts what the relationship will be. Correlational tests were discussed in detail earlier in the chapter. To review them briefly: The correlational test for interval data is the *Pearson r*. This test requires that the scores on both variables be normally distributed and on interval scales. If you have ordinal data, use the *Spearman rank correlation*; with nominal categories use *Chi-square* analysis.

Estimation of Population Parameters from Sample Data. Your hypothesis may predict a population parameter (such as the mean or variance) from the sample statistic. For instance, you might plan to use the mean IQ from a sample of registered nurses to predict the IQ of the whole population of registered nurses. An ideal estimator provides an unbiased estimate of the unknown population parameter. As such, it will correspond closely to the population value when a large number of sample estimates are averaged.

All of the descriptive statistics discussed in the previous section are examples of sample statistics that can be used to predict population parameters (means, medians, standard deviations, etc.) An individual estimate obtained from one sample, however, will not necessarily be an accurate estimate of the population parameter. It is usually necessary to take the average mean from a large number of samples to get an accurate estimate of the population mean. Since you will not usually use a large number of samples, you must establish the accuracy with which your sample statistic predicts the population parameter. This is done by the use of a *confidence interval*.

A confidence interval gives you a range of values within which the true value of the population parameter is estimated to fall. You decide in advance how confident you would like to be in your estimate (say, 95% or 99%). Then, instead of saying that the population mean is 80, you will say that you estimate the population mean to be somewhere between 75 and 83, and that you are 99% sure that your estimate is correct. The range between 75 and 83 is your confidence interval.

Confidence intervals for the mean and standard deviation can be obtained using the versatile *t* test, providing the observations come from a normally distributed population with equal variances and are measured on an interval scale. Nonparametric tests for establishing confidence intervals include Tukey's confidence interval for the median and the binomial test for the confidence intervals of quartiles.

Be Sure You Can Answer Your Question

The brief discussion of statistical analysis presented here has been for the sole purpose of guiding the beginning researcher to plan a simple analysis for a simple question. The major criterion for analysis technique is that the results provide the answer to the question. It follows from this that the researcher must understand the technique. If you choose a technique that is beyond your understanding, it will be very difficult to interpret the results of your study. It is better to be simple and sure than complex and incomprehensible.

THE ANSWER IS IN THE QUESTION

The plan for data analysis is intended to provide support for one answer rather than another to your research question. As we have stressed throughout this book, the type of answer you require depends on how you asked the question. Look again at the chart in the front of the book that outlines the three levels of studies. Now is the time to review your plan to make sure that it logically follows one of the three levels, and that the answer you have planned will be the answer to your original question. If your plan is consistent and logical, the data analysis plan will help you distinguish the best answer among the possible alternatives. So look now at your *stem question,* because it *specifies the answer* you need.

Level I Questions. Your question asked *what, where, when,* or *who.* From the data you plan to collect and the analysis you have planned, you should be able to envision what the answer will look like. You will have categories into which you can put your observations. If the question asked *who,* the categories will reflect who was in the sample. For *when* questions, the categories will describe time periods, stages, or phases. The answer can then be described from the summarization of data into categories. Conclusions from level I studies can be the development of concepts, the discovery of operational definitions, or a prediction about the relationship between categories of variables.

Level II Questions. Your question at this level asks about the relationships among variables. The answers must provide descriptions of these relationships, which must be statistically significant if the relationships are to be worth pursuing further. Therefore, level II answers must be based on statistical analysis. Conclusions drawn from level II studies include the development of hypotheses to be used in explanatory studies, and proposals for explaining the relationships among the variables using the conceptual framework of the study.

Level III Questions. Answers to level III questions depend on whether the research hypotheses were supported by the data, thus validating the theoretical or conceptual framework for the study. The framework provides the *explanation* for the action of the variables. If the question asks *why,* the answer must explicitly explain why the variables act as they do based on the theoretical framework. An *if-then* question is simpler to answer, since the prediction you have made will either occur or not occur in a statistically significant manner. But answers to *if-then* questions also must be related to the theoretical base.

Pausing now to visualize your answer will help you make sure your research plan is consistently leading you toward that answer.

RECOMMENDED READING

Conover, W. J. *Practical Non-parametric Statistics.* New York: John Wiley and Sons, 1971.

Dixon, W. J., and Massey, F. J., Jr. *Introduction to Statistical Analysis.* New York: McGraw-Hill Book Co., 1969.

Siegel, S. *Non-parametric Statistics for the Behavioral Sciences.* New York: McGraw-Hill Book Co., 1956.

XV.

From Plan to Proposal

Follow Your Outline

Fill in the Gaps

Polishing the Draft

Check Your References

The Finished Proposal

From the time you began reading this book, you read over and over again that the research plan is the most critical phase of the research process, since it forms the basis for the rest of the process. As you know, it is easier to change a plan than it is to change an almost-finished product based upon a faulty plan.

Now that you have seen all the parts to the research plan, all that is left is to write it up into a final proposal. Research and word-of-mouth are not compatible. Every part of research, from the beginning question to the final report, needs to be written down. Therefore, the research plan that is not written into a proposal is not complete.

You may be asking how we differentiate *research plan* from *research proposal* at this late date. In our opinion, the difference between the two is as great as that between your beginning working definitions and your final operational definitions. The research plan is your basic outline of your entire research idea with your bibliography cards, your working definitions, and so on. Your research proposal is your essay that fills in all of the gaps of the outline, makes all of the logical transitions for the reader, and shows the consistent development of the idea from question to answer.

The art of writing the proposal in such a way that someone else can follow your train of thought requires serious consideration. You don't want your project to be lost at this stage simply because you were inarticulate. The final step, the research proposal, is worth the effort.

FOLLOW YOUR OUTLINE

Every research proposal has a slightly different character, as you will notice when you look over the ones in the Appendix. The reason is rather basic—a research proposal reflects the personality of the writer. Although the basic parts of a proposal are identical and include every major point in chapter IV, the way in which you write each aspect of the proposal is a reflection on you.

Look at your outline again. If you haven't already done it, your first task is to write your topic as an essay called the *Research Problem* as described in chapter III. Sometimes this forces you to think about the transition between parts of the topic as outlined. Remember that there should be a rationale for the development of your question, a literature review, and a conceptual or theoretical framework upon which your study is based. All of this needs to be written in such a way that your reader follows the logic of your position.

So, following the topical outline of chapter IV, you must first write the introductory matter of the proposal—the introduction, body, and conclusion of your research problem, your purpose, and your operational definitions—in that order. The second half of your outline

is your design section. Follow the outline given in chapter IV. Begin
with what research approach you intend to use: exploratory descriptive, descriptive survey, explanatory experimental, or a combination.
Then go on to discuss the sample in detail, and describe the method or
methods of data collection you have decided to use and why. Describe
the particular tool or tools you are using, where they came from, how
they are used in this particular study, how they have been (or will be)
tested for reliability and validity. And finally, discuss which data analysis techniques you plan to use on the data, and why.

Just as chapter IV is an outline of this entire book and each
chapter follows that outline, so too will your research proposal follow
the outline you have developed from your initial research question. As
you write your proposal, make sure that you are still at the same level of
research that you started with. Look over the three levels of research
again. If you began with a level I question and stuck with it, then you
must have at least a rationale for your problem along with your literature review. Your purpose—to explore and describe a variable—must
be written as a declarative statement. Your operational definitions
must treat every variable as independent. Your design must be descriptive or exploratory; it will use open-ended questionnaires or interviews; unstructured or semi-structured observations; and, probably,
some form of available data. Your answer will describe your findings,
develop concepts, or categorize processes using content analysis,
graphs, charts, tables, or descriptive statistics.

If you began with a level II question, you know something about
your variables and are looking at the relationship between and among
them. Here you must have a conceptual framework along with your
rationale and literature review, and you should be able to operationally
define your terms with greater precision. Your research design must be
a descriptive survey design because, unlike the exploratory descriptive
design, you as the researcher have some control over the situation
under study. As a result your purpose must be written as a question.
This level of research cannot predict the action of the variables, so the
methods you use will reflect this. Interviews and questionnaires will be
structured, either open, closed or mixed. Observations must be structured and projective tests may be used. Data should be analyzed in
relation to inferential statistics, correlation analysis, and the differences between means. The answer to level II questions lies in hypothesis development or the explanation of the relationship between and
among variables in the conceptual framework. The answer will differ
from the level I question which will describe what was found, attempt
to categorize the variables and/or processes found, or develop concepts
for further testing at level II.

The level III questions are the *why* or *if-then* questions, which yield
explanatory or experimental designs. At level III, you must know

about your variables. You base your study on a conceptual or theoretical framework and *predict* the action of your variables. For this reason, you *must* write your purpose as an hypothesis. Your design, therefore, is under the control of the investigator. The *why* question yields explanations about the independent variable, whereas the if-then question yields experiments on the independent variable to explain the result in the dependent variable. Therefore, all methods and data analysis are available to do one or the other of those two things. The answer must either support or reject the hypothesis, thereby adding to the knowledge base of the conceptual or theoretical framework.

FILL IN THE GAPS

All outlines are simply a skeleton for a final paper. No outline, in and of itself, can stand alone as a finished written product. There are always gaps to be filled in. Notice how the outline in chapter II was translated into an essay in chapter III. The essay made the connections between the ideas in the outline. Filling in the gaps in the outline constitutes writing the essay, and involves nothing more than forming the ideas in the outline into paragraphs and linking them with transition sentences.

If you have difficulty in writing, there are several books on the market that can help you. You have already been referred to Payne in chapter II for writing the introductory matter. The references at the end of chapter II are also excellent.

POLISHING THE DRAFT

The difference between a first draft of a research proposal and the final polished draft is enormous and generally reflects the amount of time between the first written draft and the final polished proposal.

Students usually have a limited amount of time between learning to write a proposal, and all of the steps involved in the research process, and actually submitting that proposal. As a result, the product submitted is often a first draft—rough, awkward and sometimes almost inarticulate.

To minimize these defects, we suggest that a friend review the first draft before you submit it to the instructor. Have the friend describe the project. This will tell you if the proposal is clear and logical. On the basis of this initial critique; changes should be made in the paper prior to submitting it. If your friend doesn't understand what you are doing, the possibility exists that your instructor won't either.

If you possibly can, put your first draft of the proposal away and let it "sit" for a while. Don't take it out again for at least two weeks, preferrably two months. You will be amazed at what happens to your thinking when you let your project sit long enough so that you can see what you have written with a critical analytical eye—not the eye of a fond parent. Your mistakes will loom clearly before you—how your sentences seem muddy, your logic not apparent, your idea not communicated. Now you are ready to polish the first draft. This is simply a matter of rewriting. Now is the time to clarify your ideas, write transition sentences, make the tense consistent, clean up typographical errors, and so on. You may end up revising the entire proposal, but better that than having it turned down because it failed to communicate your ideas.

CHECK YOUR REFERENCES

When you write a research proposal, you are expected to be accurate in all details—major and minor. But most important is to be accurate in your referencing. Nothing is worse, especially in research, than misquoting, misreferencing, or failing to give proper credit. You never know if the author of a research report upon which you based your ideas will be reading your proposal.

Unfortunately, human beings are not computers—we all have a tendency to make errors. To be sure that you have listed all the references cited in the body of the paper, reread your entire proposal just for the references, and check each one against your list. Time-consuming? Yes. Worth it? Definitely. You never know when you may need that exact, correct reference.

THE FINISHED PROPOSAL

The finished proposal should have a sense of closure, of completeness about it. All parts are present and accounted for—including the title page.

Completed proposals look good. They are typed, double-spaced, and have page numbers. Handwritten proposals simply are not acceptable, nor are proposals that have been edited so much that they are practically handwritten. Clean, neat proposals are not just pleasing to the eye; they create a positive impression on the reader. But don't let typographical errors stand uncorrected in the final copy simply to preserve the whiteness of the sheet. By all means correct your typos. If you have too many, retype the page. The use of liquid paper has become a boon to people who don't type professionally.

Your finished proposal, hopefully less than 25 typed pages in length, is what you will present to your instructor at the end of the course; submit to a committee for the protection of human rights; use as the basis for any grant proposal you may decide to write later; and use as a guide for the rest of the research process. Since it serves so many functions, make more than one copy of the proposal. Consider how you would feel if it were lost. Also make sure that everything you may need to refer to in your future research is included in the proposal, since that is probably all you will be referring to, rather than your stacks of notes and bibliography cards. If you keep the uses of the proposal in mind, you may consider that brevity is a virtue—and indeed it is. Be as brief as possible without losing your train of thought or neglecting an important point.

Type the final proposal on bonded paper that has some cotton content so the words will not smudge. If you use corrasible bond, the paper not only sticks to your hands (and everyone else's), but smudges every time you touch the type. So use a durable bond paper and erase with liquid paper. If you do, your proposal will last until the end of the project and beyond.

On your final check of the finished proposal, delete all personal nouns and pronouns. Everyone knows this is your proposal, so referring to yourself is simply redundant. But if you must, use the third person—call yourself the researcher or investigator.

As you write up your proposal, try to remember that what you are writing about is what you intend to do in the future. Therefore, your proposal should be written in future tense. Write clearly, with as little superfluity, pomposity, and garrulousness as possible. Some people feel that a scholarly proposal is unintelligible to the general reader. This does not have to be true. Write it so *you* can understand it; when you read it a month or two later, you will remember what you were thinking about, and can go on from there.

The finished research paper, whether written by one person or a group, is a reflection of the time and thinking that went into the plan from question to proposal. The finished proposal marks the end of one phase of research—it is a milestone achieved.

Appendixes

Glossary

Clinical Nursing Research: Distinguished from Nursing Research by the topic under study. Generally agreed to be primarily involved with direct nurse-patient interactions. May focus secondarily on either nursing practice as it ultimately affects nurse/patient interactions, or on the patient as having an ultimate effect on nurse/patient interactions.

Components of the Question: Refers to the basic parts of the research question—the stem and the topic.

Concept: A single idea, usually a single word, that represents at least two related component ideas.

Conceptual Framework: The use of one or more concepts as the rationale beind the selection of the problem for study. When one concept is used, the component or interconnecting ideas within the concept are discussed as the basis for the study. Or the concept is discussed in relationship to the variables to be studied. When two or more concepts are linked together to explain the topic, then the relationship between and among the concepts related to the problem forms the conceptual framework.

Convenience Sample: A nonprobability sample, chosen for their accessibility to the researcher. Also called an available sample.

Construct: A concept that has been invented or adopted for a special purpose, e.g., to explain or test a concept under study. Usually a higher level of abstraction and further removed from being directly observed than a concept.

Data Analysis: A systematic method for arranging and describing the data or statistical testing of hypotheses on which to base inferences.

Definition of Terms: All words used in the final stated purpose of the study are described in relation to what is meant by the word for the study and how the word will be studied. Usually a separate part of the research plan in the introductory matter prior to the discussion on design.

Dependent Variable: A variable that results from the action of another; the effect of a change in an independent variable. *See also* Independent Variable.

Experimental Explanatory Design: Design in which all variables are controlled by the researcher during the data collection phase, including the sample. Always based on an if-then question. Data analysis utilizes statistics and draws inferences.

Explanatory Design: *See* Experimental Explanatory Design; Explanatory Survey Design.

Explanatory Survey Design: Design that uses data collection and data analysis to explain the relationship between two or more variables. Based upon *why* question. This design does not impose an independent variable on the sample.

Extraneous Variable: Any variable that might effect the outcome of a study but is not of immediate or direct interest to the researcher. These variables may alter the presumed association between independent and dependent variables, if they have not been controlled by the research design.

Fact: Any thing or idea that is *accepted* as true.

Hypothesis: A specific statement of relationship between two or more variables, based upon a conceptual or theoretical framework. Often a statement of causal relationships between an independent and dependent variable, or a statement of the precise association between variables. Must be based upon prior research in the area and knowledge of the characteristics of the variables used.

Independent Variable: A variable that stands alone. Comes first in time, or is assumed to cause a change in another variable. The variable manipulated or altered by the researcher. Also called the experimental variable, or the cause. *See also* Dependent Variable.

Instruments: Tools or devices used to collect data for a study.

Interval Scale: Scale with an arbitrary zero point and numerically equal distances between points on the scale. There is a zero point which has been arbitrarily placed on the scale. Because the intervals are equal, they can be added and subtracted. For example on a scale of

0–20, the intervals from 2 to 5 represent the same amount of the characteristic being measured as do the intervals from 10 to 13. However, because the zero point is arbitrary, it is not possible to say that a score of ten represents twice as much of the characteristic as does a score of five. Thermometers and IQ tests are interval scales.

Measurement Definitions: Refers to the definition of terms at the early stages of research planning in which every word in the research question must be defined in such a way that the word can be counted, observed or measured in some way.

Methods: Specific procedures by which the sample and the data from the sample will be collected according to the research design chosen.

Model: A graph, diagram, chart, or verbal outline of a concept or theory showing the interrelationships of the parts to the whole.

Nominal Scale: Two or more mutually-exclusive categories into which objects, events, or people can be classified. No magnitude or value difference exists between the categories. For example: sex—male/female; religion—Protestant/Catholic/Buddhist.

Nonprobability Sample: A sample deliberately selected to meet the need of the study.

Nursing Research: Research involved with nursing issues—clinical nursing topics, nursing processes and functions, the nursing profession, or nursing knowledge.

Observation: A sensory experience (looking, listening, tasting, smelling, feeling) that can be described specifically for research.

Operational Definition: A full and complete description of what and how one variable will be studied. Includes all components of the variable to be studied and the method of examining that variable.

Ordinal Scale: Two or more categories arranged in increasing or decreasing order to which has been attached some value or magnitude. Also meets assumptions of nominal scale with added dimension of attaching value to each category. Example: poor/fair/good; ugly/ordinary/beautiful; strongly agree/agree/disagree/strongly disagree. Although these categories are arranged in order on some continuum, the precise distance between the points on the scale cannot be measured.

Population: The universe of people, things or events about which the research is involved. Has specific characteristics required for the research; serves as the basis for sample selection.

Principle: A statement of the relationship between facts that is *accepted* as true and used as the basis for explaining phenomena.

Probability Sample: Sample for which every member of the target population for the research study has a known chance of being selected.

Problem-Solving: The use of the scientific process to resolve an immediate crisis or difficulty. Usually specific to a single area, a single problem, or a single sample. Not generalizable beyond the sample.

Program Evaluation: An applied research method specifically testing the effectiveness of one program. Usually the research involves testing the method by which the program is meeting its stated objectives.

Purpose: A statement of *what* or who the researcher intends to study, *where* it is to be done, and *on whom* the study is to be done. Specifies the research problem into one specific study; is written as statement, question, or hypothesis.

Quota Sample: A nonprobability sample selected to represent certain characteristics in the population as a whole. When a particular population (whether people, animals, events or things) has specific chracteristics that the investigator wishes to have represented in the study, then the sample must be selected on the basis of these characteristics. Such a sample must also indicate the minimum versus the maximum number needed to represent that characteristic. A nonprobability sample.

Ratio Scales: Meets all criteria for an interval scale with an absolute zero point. The point on the scale where none of the characteristics is present is known. Therefore, all arithmetic operations are possible. On a yardstick measuring height 6 feet is twice as large as 3 feet. On a scale measuring weight, 25 pounds is one fourth as heavy as 100 pounds. Many physiological and biochemical measurements such as blood pressure, pulse, blood counts, and body chemistries are ratio scales.

Research: A systematized method for gaining new knowledge that can be verified and generalized beyond the sample studied.

Research Design: A "blueprint for action"; the overall general categories that describe the conditions under which the data will be collected and analyzed to accomplish the purpose of the study. Always includes methods of both data collection and analysis of data.

Research Problem: A logical discussion of the situation, idea, concept, or theory that prompted the study. Provides frame of reference for the purpose, places the study in a context of related research and thinking. Establishes the rationale for the level of research (descriptive or explanatory).

Research Proposal: A written plan of what is to be studied, how the study will be conducted, how the data will be analyzed, and the rationale for the project.

Research Question: A *what, where, when, who, why, if-then* question asked of the research topic.

Research Topic: The subject, idea, concept, or theory to be studied. Answers the questions: What do you really want to know? What do you really want to study?

Sample: The specific group of people, things, or events to be included in a research study. Must represent or be characteristic of the population from which it is drawn. Size depends on the research topic, the population from which it is drawn, and the purpose of the study.

Stem Question: The words preceding the research topic. Usually includes *what, when, where, why, who, if-then.*

Stratified Random Sample: A randomly selected probability sample of groups, each of which represents a certain characteristic of the population.

Target Population: *See* Population.

Theoretical Framework: The use of one theory or interrelated theories to support the rationale behind a study.

Theory: An idea, often stated in a single word or short phrase, that represents the relationship between two or more concepts. Unlike a concept, they require a full and complete explanation of conceptual interaction.

Variable: Any thing, event, or person that can be measured or described on some scale; anything that varies or qualitatively alters along some dimension.

Working Definition: The researcher's beginning description of the situation, variables, concepts, or theories to be tested in the research. The definition is based on the researcher's own frame of reference at the time of writing the research question. Usually an attempt to describe what is to be studied in some form of measurement, or scale. A working definition differs from an operational definition in relation to its lack of statement of how the variable is to be studied, and lack of precision in relation to research literature.

Sample Research Proposals

The samples of proposals in the following pages are not perfect, nor do they all meet all of the requirements of a proper proposal as discussed throughout this book. They are, however, clear and logical, and give some idea of the format to follow. With one exception, they were written by students as a first effort for their first research course. The criteria for selection of these proposals was relatively simple—first we asked if these research plans could actually be carried out; second, if they reflected different approaches to nursing research; third, if they represented different ideas or topics; and fourth, if they were brief enough for inclusion. (Some were edited for brevity, others were brief to begin with.) All lists of references were deliberately deleted as not exemplifying the style of writing a proposal. Methods of referencing can be found elsewhere.

DOES THE EDUCATIONAL LEVEL EFFECT THE NURSE'S ROLE PERCEPTION AND JOB SATISFACTION?

by Mary E. McClelland

Introduction

As a result of the 1965 American Nurses' Association position paper on nursing education, nurses from four different educational levels are now practicing in health care agencies. The position paper identified three essential components of professional nursing. These three components, care, cure, and coordination, were utilized as a basis in the proposed educational preparation of the baccalaureate degree, the associate degree, and the licensed vocational nurse.

The conceptual framework of this study includes the perceptions that graduate nurses of baccalaureate degree, associate degree, diploma, and licensed vocational programs have of their role. Using the components of professional nursing, care, cure, and coordination, the role perceptions of these four levels of nurses will be studied in relation to their job satisfaction.

Purpose

The purpose of this study is to answer the two questions:

1. Is there a difference in the perception of a nurse's role based on the educational preparation of the nurse?

2. Is there a difference in the job satisfaction of these different levels of nurses?

Definition of Terms

Educational level—the type of preparatory program from which the nurse received her original education in nursing.

Baccalaureate Degree Nurse—a graduate of a collegiate nursing program with a bachelor of science degree in nursing.

Associate Degree Nurse—a graduate of a junior college program with an associate degree in nursing.

Diploma Nurse—a graduate of a hospital-based training program.

Licensed Vocational Nurse—a graduate of a vocational training program.

Written as a graduate student research proposal for the Committee on the Protection of Human Rights. Footnotes deleted. By Permission of the Author.

Role Perception—the interpretations the individual makes of the expected functions of a position.

Job Satisfaction—the attitude the individual develops of the position in which he functions within the organization.

Research Design

To study perceptions, a descriptive survey design will be used. A questionnaire will be used to collect data from the subjects.

Sample and Setting

A sample of licensed vocational, diploma, associate degree, and baccalaureate degree nurses will be chosen from three hospitals of over 250 beds within the Los Angeles area. The subjects must have completed their original educational program within the last two years. The subjects from each institution will be chosen randomly from the entire licensed vocational and registered nurse population who have completed their original nursing education within the last two years.

The subject's consent will be granted by the completion and return of the questionnaire. A cover letter will accompany each questionnaire explaining this and the study.

Data Collection Instrument

A questionnaire developed by the investigator using an Osgood semantic differential scale will be used to obtain data on the attitudes the nurses have towards nursing functions. These nursing functions will represent the care, cure, and coordination aspects of professional nursing practice.

Data on job satisfaction will be obtained by using the Smith Job Descriptive Index.

Data Collection Method

The Director of Nursing of each of the three institutions will be contacted for permission to conduct the study within the institution. Any other institutional requirements will also be followed.

Each subject will be chosen randomly from the total population of registered nurses and licensed vocational nurses meeting the requirements of the study. After the study group is chosen they will receive their questionnaire by mail and will be asked to return it by mail. Each questionnaire will contain a letter explaining the study and asking for their consent by completing the questionnaire.

Analysis of Data

Inferential statistics will be used to analyze the difference in attitudes between the four different levels of nurses in relation to their role perceptions in care, cure, and coordination.

A parametric F test will be used to test for a significant difference between the four groups.

LIFE ENERGY OR ELECTRICAL ARTIFACT?

by Lori Mennen

Introduction

"In the recorded and prerecorded history of many civilizations around the world, there can be found a powerful tradition of invisible energy of fluid which interpenetrates the universe. This energy has been given various names in various cultures. The ancient Egyptians called it *Ka*, the Hindus and Yogis, *Prana*, the Chinese, *Chi*, and the Hawaiians, *Mana*. Whatever the name, this invisible energy has existed and been written about."

Since the 1890's many have attempted to develop a special type of photographic process which shows on film thi; invisible energy. However, it wasn't until 1939 that two Soviet research scientists, Semyon and Valentina Kirlian, began experimenting with contact photography in a high-frequency field. They published several articles about this process in Soviet technical journals in 1959. This information was made available to the American public in the early 1970's.

Investigators discovered that the photographic process developed by the Kirlians is referred to by several names: Kirlian photography, electrophotography, radiation field photography, or coronal discharge photography. These names evolved from the different theories that attempt to explain the energy photography.

It has been speculated that the energy revealed by the Kirlian photographic process may be a direct measure of life activities occurring within a living organism. Based on this speculation, some see

---

By permission of the author. Footnotes deleted.

Kirlian photographs as having an array of possibilities as a medical diagnostic tool. In the U.S.S.R., Kirlian photographs are said to be used in cancer research.

The Problem

"Cancer cells can arise in any body tissue at any age. Characteristically, the cells can invade local tissues by direct extension or they can spread throughout the body by way of the lymphatic or vascular channels."

The American Cancer Society estimates that more than one million Americans will be under medical care for cancer in 1976. 675,000 of the one million will be newly diagnosed. It has also, been estimated that 370,000 people will die of cancer (202,000 males and 168,000 females).

In 1976, approximately 93,000 people will be stricken with cancer of the respiratory system and 88,450 of these people will die (68,900 males and 19,550 females). Cancer of the respiratory system includes the larynx, lung, and other unspecified respiratory components.

Specifically, lung cancer is a largely preventable disease, since it is mainly caused by cigarette smoking. Unfortunately, it is difficult to diagnose in time for a cure. Only about ten percent of the reported cases are being saved.

Kirlian photography may be the diagnostic tool that can perform this lifesaving task. Some studies exemplify this: Moss (1976) carried on a study involving two hundred rats. She regularly found that the tail of a healthy rat showed a full emanation while the tumerous rats showed a photograph of a tail with "crud" (crud is an irregular emanation from a central source).

Hubacher (1976) carried out a double blind study with serum from patients with cancer of the head and neck. He applied three to five drops of serum on a cover slip, then using the Kirlian process, took photographs. These results revealed no gross differences.

Gorgshein and Traister performed a study using cancerous whole blood. He had been taking Kirlian photographs of whole clotted blood in test tubes without any additives and whole blood drawn up in pipettes from patients with cancer. The blood drawn up in pipettes was centrifuged for five minutes and the serum removed. He used black and white film paper made by Kodak. His population consisted of six patients of different ages with varying types of cancer and one normal blood sample. The results revealed gross differences. The normal blood sample had a small sparse emanation as compared to the cancerous blood samples with emanations that were prominent and continuous. The photographed serum showed the opposite.

Purpose of Study

The purpose of this investigation is to determine if the difference between Kirlian photographs of blood samples in men ages 21 to 75 is effective in the diagnosis of cancer of the respiratory system. The assumption made is that when cancer is present in the respiratory system, it is also present in the blood.

Definition of Terms

1. *Kirlian photograph:* the image or picture produced on a film negative that shows an emanation or discharge radiating out from a central source in a 360 degree form.

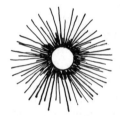

This photographed emanation will be measured for:
    a) The total length of the emanation in millimeters.

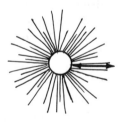

    b) Number of layers.

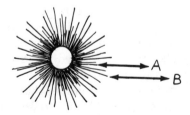

   c) Gapping distance in millimeters.

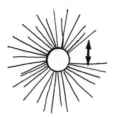

   d) Density as measured by a spectrometer by percent of transmission of light.
   e) Bubbles measured by absence given a value of 1 or presence given a value of 2.

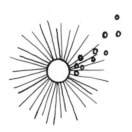

2. *Blood Sample:* 1-2cc of human blood (unoxygenated) from the vein and left unrefrigerated for not more than 24 hours in a test tube containing an anticoagulant.

3. *Cancer in Whole Blood (experimental group):* presence of recognizable histopathological (abnormal cell) changes that occur with cancer which are found in the respiratory system and can be detected by a microscopic examination by trained laboratory personnel. The whole blood will be measured by Kirlian photographs in terms of density, number of layers, length of emanation, gapping distance, and bubbles.

4. *No Cancer in Whole Blood (control group):* no recognizable histopathological changes that occur with cancer cells in the respiratory system. The blood obtained is from a person who has no history of any other type of cancer present on or in the body. This whole blood will be measured by Kirlian photographs in terms of density, number of layers, length of emanation, gapping distance, and bubbles.

Research Approach

The design of this study is methodological. The development of a new tool always requires a serious, well-controlled study. It must be determined that the tool is providing genuine information or if the information is distorted by its own technology. This study will be testing the

Kirlian tool for reliability and validity. This will be accomplished by comparing the photographs of blood from persons with and without cancer to see if this tool can detect a difference.

According to Moss/Hubacher/Johnson, "it was a long time before artifacts (or changed appearances produced by the tool itself) were isolated from the EEG, GSR, EKG, and a host of other electrical equipment. . . ." "The artifact controversy has just begun with Kirlian photography. . . ." "Some enthusiasts claim this electrical photography reveals the human aura (life energies), while the conservatives maintain the photographs reveal a commonplace electrical phenomenon frequently seen when high voltage is passed through a wire."

In most instances, Kirlian photographs cannot be obtained unless a jolt of high voltage (a high potential of force which can alter the motion of electricity) and low ampherage (strength of an electric current) is sent through the object being photographed. However, this theory has been questioned when Moss found that by pressing a human fingertip on undeveloped film, then developing the film while the finger is held in place, that a dim emanation was visible with some people.

"Nevertheless, electricity is an important ingredient. Therefore, what is revealed in a photograph must be in part due to the frequency (the number of cycles per second of an alternating current), pulse (rhythm of the current), voltage, and duration of electrical flow. What is produced on film is clearly a function of those electrical parameters and may be the result of artifact. However there are abnormalities."

Moss has found unusual differences which can not be explained by electrical artifact as we know it. Several examples used concern the photographs of plant leaves:

1. Kirlian photographs reveal each variety of leaf has its own special emanation with bubbles. Plant biologists have informed her that the surface characteristics of the leaf particularly the bubbles have no physiological or anatomical correlation.

2. She found if the same leaf was photographed over a period of days its picture changed from bright to dim. The leaf itself remained physically intact and fresh to touch. This held true with Hubacher's photographs of whole blood taken over a period of several days. The emanation became increasingly dim.

3. There is also the phantom leaf effect. Part of a leaf (2–10%) is removed and then the leaf is immediately photographed. On the developed film was the emanation of a whole leaf. This missing part was reconstructed in the picture!

4. Moss has also discovered unusual phenomena occurring in the developed photographs of fingertips showing interactions between people, emotional states, healing, and intoxication with alcohol and marijuana vs. sober states.

Electrical artifact or life energy, whatever the emanations represent, certain changes have been observed to occur. These changes demonstrate a challenge to the psychological and medical fields. Obviously, only preliminary studies have been made. More well-controlled studies with replications of each are essential to discover the true reliability and validity of this tool.

The Pretest. A pretest will be performed prior to the actual study. It will involve ten males: five with cancer of the respiratory system and five without. Blood will be obtained from the above-mentioned using the described double blind system. The samples used in the pretest will not be used in the actual study.

The Sample. A selected sample will be used in this study. The samples of whole blood will be given to the researcher from M. Cline, U.C.L.A. Cancer Research Laboratory, B. Dettmar, U.C.L.A. Clinical Laboratory, and A. Fisher, UCLA Oncology Clinic, based on the following criteria: the blood will be obtained from males between the ages of 21–75 with the diagnosis of cancer vs. no cancer (see definition of terms). The demographic characteristics to be considered are: age, sex, and medical diagnosis. Everything else will be considered as extraneous variables.

Data Collection. It will be a double blind study to prevent the investigator's biases from interfering with the photographic process. This will be accomplished by obtaining mixed whole blood samples from the Cancer Research Laboratory and clinical laboratories which will have numerically coded labels. A value of *1* will be given for cancer and *2* for no cancer. These labels will be covered. The investigator will take Kirlian photographs of forty whole blood samples: twenty from males with cancer of the respiratory system and twenty without cancer. The cover will be removed from the test tube after the picture has been taken and analyzed.

The setting for this study will be the Parapsychology Laboratory in the NPI building at UCLA, (28–181). This setting was selected for three reasons:

a) use of one of the Kirlian instruments in the isolation chamber (a metal chamber in which Kirlian instruments are set up as well as equipment for developing film).

b) geographical proximity to UCLA School of Nursing.

c) availability of blood samples in close proximity to the Parapsychology Laboratory so it will remain fresh and viable.

Four months will be allowed for the completion of this study. The first month will be used to complete a pretest of the Kirlian instrument. The last three months will be used to collect data for investigation including obtaining blood samples, taking photographs, and developing the film.

The Kirlian Technique

1. *Kirlian instrument.* I will be using an instrument developed by K. Johnson. It is a modification of an instrument he devised earlier and is discussed in Johnson's book, *The Living Aura.* The instrument consists of three units: the generation of electrical parameters, conducting area, and the ground. The generation of the electrical parameters consists of six instruments. They are:

a) *power source*—a high voltage power supply. It consists of a step up transformer. A transformer is an apparatus that transforms voltages of an electric current. The step-up transformer changes low voltage into high voltage. Type model used is in-house built.

b) *push-button oscillator*—instrument that causes change in the direction or variation between maximum (positive) and minimum (negative) values in voltage or current. It gives the voltage a cycle or frequency. The type of instrument used is Krohn-Hite Model 440 A.

c) *ROB counter*—reads the actual frequencies being emitted. Type instrument used is Dymec Model 25038.

d) *pulse generator*—takes the frequency and pulses it or emits voltage of current at specifically determined intervals. The type of instrument used is Rutherford Model B7B.

e) *Oscilloscope*—visually records an electrical wave on a flourescent screen. It allows one to measure frequency, voltage and ampheres. Type instrument used is Hewitt-Packard Co. Model 6625–989–5448.

The conducting area consists of:

a) a capacitor—a plate that receives and stores an electrical charge. It is made of carbon steel, and is approximately 4″ × 6″.

b) dielectric—a sheet of thin plastic which prevents the conduction of electrical current.

c) the unexposed film (Tri-X black-and-white film made by Kodak). Tri-X is used for high film speeds and fast exposure. It is a more sensitive type of film. The exposure time will be 1/30 second.

d) coverslip with blood—3 gtts. of blood will be placed on coverslip of a 4 thickness.

The ground consists of:

a) ground (+)—electricity doesn't flow unless it goes from a higher to lower voltage. The lower voltage is called the ground area.

The following is a diagram of the entire unit:

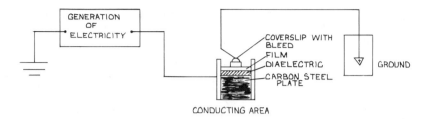

An object (the blood) is placed on an electrically charged plate (capacitor) next to a piece of unexposed film. When the plate is electrically activated an electrostatic field is established and the object being photographed becomes charged. The photographic film next to the object automatically receives a discharge from the object that forms a latent image on film which can be developed into a visable negative image.

All pictures will be taken in a metal isolation chamber where the photographic equipment is set up. The temperature range is 70–80 degrees farenheit. This chamber is also used as the darkroom to develop the film negative. A standard brand of print developer, called Dektol (made by Kodak), is used. It is basically alkaline in nature and it turns the photographed image black. The exposed film is left in the Dektol for 1–2 minutes. The exposed film is then transferred to a fixer solution called Naccofix (made by Kodak). Its entire function is to stop development of the film. It is acid in nature. The exposed film is left in the Naccofix for approximately 3 minutes. Both Dektol and Naccofix are kept in plastic pans side by side in isolation chamber. After this process is completed the negative is rinsed with tap water and allowed to air dry.

Data Analysis

In this study inferential parametric statistics will be used. The main purpose of inferential statistics is to test a research hypothesis by testing a statistical hypothesis. The use of an inferential (statistical) test implies the presence of the null hypothesis. The null hypothesis is a statistical proposition which states essentially a zero relation between variables.

A one-way analysis of variance will be used. It is a method of identifying, breaking down, and testing data for statistical significance. This method maintains the precision of measurements and prevents the discarding of potentially valuable data. The following is a diagram which identifies and breaks down data that will be used:

independent variables: A_1 = cancer A_2 = no cancer

dependent variable: B_1 = total length of emanations in millimeters

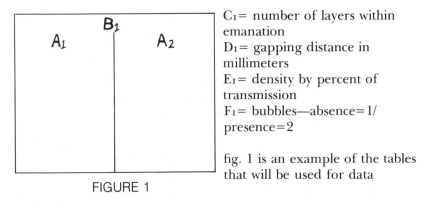

C_1 = number of layers within emanation
D_1 = gapping distance in millimeters
E_1 = density by percent of transmission
F_1 = bubbles—absence = 1/ presence = 2

fig. 1 is an example of the tables that will be used for data

FIGURE 1

To test for statistical significance, an f-ratio will be used. It is computed using the following formula: $\dfrac{\text{variance between groups}}{\text{variance within groups}}$

After the f-ratio is calculated, the results are checked against an f-table. If the obtained f-ratio is as great or greater than the appropriate table entry, the differences that the variance between reflects are statistically significant. In such a case the null hypothesis of no differences between the means is rejected at the chosen level of significance.

Limitations of the Study

Three categories must be considered:

1. Limitations within the Kirlian process as variations in voltage, ampherage, pulse duration, unequal pressures of blood on the film, uneven chemical distribution on the film itself, the frequency of exposure time, distance the object is placed from the film.

2. Limitations due to environmental conditions such as variations in room temperature, wind currents in chamber, changes in posture of the person taking the photographs.

3. Limitations due to conditions within the patient as use of drugs, radiation treatment, presence of other diseases in the body, blood type, race, age, emotional state of the patient at time blood drawn, or after the patient has eaten.

It would be extremely difficult to control for all of the above-mentioned due to the amount of time allotted for this study, the researchers' limited knowledge, and limited knowledge of the Kirlian instrument itself.

These limitations will obviously have some affect on the applicability of the findings and will be considered when the product of data analysis is obtained. These limitations will need further research in terms of reliability and validity of the tool before conclusive evidence may be significantly stated.

This study is not meant to unlock the mysterious hieroglyphics of the Kirlian photographs, but to assist in the building of a strong foundation for which other studies may be continued.

Protection of Human Rights

According to Notter there are three factors involved in the protection of the rights of individuals used as subjects of research:

1. *Informed consent.* The blood samples will be obtained from the UCLA Cancer Research Laboratory. The purpose, procedures, risks, and potential benefits of this activity will be explained to the above-mentioned laboratory and hospital administrator.

2. *Confidentiality of the data collected.* According to the established investigation, the researcher will not at any time know the patient's name. Only the sex, age, and medical diagnosis will be made available. No medical records will be reviewed. These measures will provide for complete confidentiality and not invade the privacy of the patients whose blood samples were used.

3. *Protection of the individual from harm.* The patient will not at any time be exposed to physical, psychological, or social stress due to this research. No direct or indirect coercion or perceived loss of access to health care exists. Only available adult blood samples from the previously mentioned laboratory will be used and there will be no financial remuneration for participation in this study.

DIFFERENCES IN LIFE CHANGE EVENTS AMONG RELAPSED AND UNRELAPSED EX-HEROIN ADDICTS

by Ellen Neiman

Statement of the Problem

To date, no studies have been published which explore the factors which effect relapse into heroin addiction after prolonged periods of abstinence. Considering the high recidivism rates after graduation from drug abuse treatment programs—which are in the nature of

---

Written as a final paper for the first course in research by Ellen Neiman, graduate student, UCLA School of Nursing, fall quarter 1976. Footnotes, questionnaires, and appendixes deleted. By permission of the author.

undocumented common knowledge—the absence of investigations of this kind by professionals in the field is noteworthy. Some researchers who have done long-term follow-up studies of addicts mention the high incidence of relapse, but there appears to be a reluctance at this point in time to acknowledge the magnitude of the problem (Vaillant, 1966a, 1966b, and 1973; O'Donnell, 1964; Levy, 1972). Avram Goldstein stands quite apart from other investigators—most of whom evaluate treatment of addicts by examining cost/benefit ratios, program attrition and retention rates, and outcomes during or immediately after treatment—when he states, "The prevention of relapse is the central challenge in the treatment of heroin addiction. Were it not for the relapse phenomenon, we could eliminate the heroin problem in a few weeks by detoxifying all the addicts," (Goldstein, 1975, p. 34).

Although workers in the drug abuse field argue incessantly about the fine points of treatment outcomes and how to measure them, and about the most effective treatment modality (methadone maintenance versus the therapeutic community versus outpatient counseling with or without initial hospital detoxification versus compulsory supervision by parole or probation officer), there is universal agreement that being unaddicted is a better state of affairs than being addicted. Addiction means shortened life expectancy, disturbed social relationships, local and systemic infectious diseases, prostitution and criminal behavior, birth of addicted infants with higher morbidity and mortality rates, inability to hold a job. Absence of addiction means refraining from criminal activity and therefore reducing the burden on both the individual and the community, doing productive work, feeling somatically well, being relieved of depression, establishing meaningful relationships and attachments with others. The goal of treatment is to free the heroin addict of psychological and physiological dependence on the drug, for his/her own welfare and that of the community at large. Recidivism, therefore, is costly to the individual and to the society.

Statistics on recidivism, or relapse, are scarce; those that exist are obfuscated by widely varying methods of measurement and minimized by manipulation of the data in order to keep a program funded or to reaffirm the obvious: being heroin-free for a period of time, however short or long, is better than not at all. Workers in the field tend to accept, somewhat fatalistically, the notion that few ex-addicts remain abstinent permanently. A high percentage of addicted individuals who have gone through the difficulties of withdrawal or detoxification, who have participated in treatment programs, and who have been abstinent for a year or more, begin to use heroin again on a regular basis at least once a day. The acceptance of this phenomenon as part of the natural history of addiction helps people in therapeutic roles to assist relapsed addicts without permitting their own judgmental attitudes to interfere in the treatment process. However, acceptance of the problem and the addict without censure does not preclude some preliminary thinking about the genesis of relapse.

Brecher writes of an intermittent anxiety, depression, and craving for heroin, described by addicts as coming and going in varying waves of intensity for as long as years after withdrawal (Brecher, 1972, p. 15). Wikler attributes the need for a "fix" and relapse long after detoxification to reactivation by previously conditioned exteroceptive and/or interoceptive stimuli. He hypothesizes that reactivation of neural processes underlying both classical and operant conditioning contributes to continued drug-seeking behavior (Wikler, 1973, p. 612).

This study will begin to explore the role of "external stressful circumstances," mentioned briefly by Goldstein (1975, p. 34), in relapse into heroin addiction. It will begin to investigate factors which effect recidivism by taking a first look at the association between stressful circumstances and relapse. The differences between these circumstances or events in the lives of ex-addicts who relapse and those who do not, during their periods of abstinence, will be examined.

Conceptual Framework and Rationale for the Study

In the course of a lifetime, everyone is exposed, to a greater or lesser extent, to widely varied situations and/or stimuli, which include life experiences such as marriage, death of a loved one, and Christmastime. Although no one has as yet attempted to make any associations between these kinds of situations and substance abuse, a growing cohort of researchers has been exploring the relationship of life's natural events to somatic and psychiatric disorders and to problems in daily living for the past three decades.

Since Selye and Wolff's early work on physiological reactions to stressors and the development by Selye and Langer and Michael of the concept of life events which produce biological and psychological changes, stressful life experiences have been linked to heart disease, fractures, childhood leukemia, tuberculosis, skin disease, beginning of prison term, poor teacher performance, low college grade point average, depression, and the common cold (Holmes and Masuda, 1974). Hinkle states, ". . . there would probably be no aspects of human growth, development, or disease that would in theory be immune to the influence of the effect of man's relation to his social and interpersonal environment" (1974, p. 10).

It is fairly clear at this point in time that stressful events play a role in adaptation and illness. The precise role that they play and the ways in which that role is mediated by physiological, psychological, and social factors have received little attention. As yet, competing hypotheses have not been generated and tested. Disagreement exists in the field about exactly how and what to measure.

A major issue in current research is the advisability of focusing on situations requiring adaptation of the organism regardless of their personal and social desirability versus those which are experienced as distressing or threatening. For most of us, a stressful event is defined in the latter terms, and some research indicates that these events are indeed the crucial one (Gersten, et al., 1974). However, the majority of studies to date have adhered to the early theories and have investigated events that change a person's life, whether the change appears to be for the better or for the worse. Holmes and Rahe, and others (e.g., Dohrenwend, 1974), use *life changes* as their domain of possibly stressful events. This approach implies that the significance of stressful events is that they require adaptation, which can mean a direct biological response that is costly to the organism, or that they involve new demands, changes in routine, and breaks in established patterns of living, with concomitant psychological threats and the need for new ways of coping (Mechanic, 1974).

Although the occurence of stressful situations or events has been shown to increase prior to the onset of many conditions, as yet no investigation has been made into the part they play in heroin addiction relapse, and more specifically, the differences in their occurence, if any, among relapsed and unrelapsed ex-addicts. This study will focus on significant life changes of all kinds, rather than on those that are viewed as threatening or distressing, since the events which flow from freedom from addiction and re-entry into the mainstream of society generally are seen as personally rewarding and positive experiences. Resumption of sexual activity, good health, the end of involvement with law enforcement agencies and the judiciary, and being able to think clearly again about something besides the next "fix" are reasons frequently given for wanting to "kick." How stressful these events are for the ex-addict is a matter for exploration as well as conjecture.

Purpose of the Study

The purpose of this study is to answer the question, Is there a difference in life change events during the period of abstinence in relapsed and unrelapsed ex-heroin addicts who have been "clean" for at least one year?

Definition of Terms

1. *Life change events:* the domain of experiences which are tem-

poral in their occurrence, as opposed to genetic or acquired constitutional endowment or developmental factors such as early mother-child relationships or a background of socio-economic deprivation. Life change events (LCE) will be measured by the Schedule of Recent Experiences (SRE) and the Social Readjustment Rating Questionnaire (SRRQ) of Holmes and Rahe, modified and adjusted for a population of heroin addicts and ex-addicts.

2. *Modified SRE-SRRQ:* a list of life change events, each of which has a numerical value called a Life Change Unit (LCU), which will be administered to all subjects in the two samples of the study—relapsed and unrelapsed ex-heroin addicts.

3. *Period of abstinence:* time period during which an individual, formerly addicted to heroin, is productively employed; not abusing narcotics, alcohol, barbiturates, tranquilizers, other central nervous system depressants, hallucinogens, or central nervous system stimulants; not on methadone maintenance; and refraining from criminal activity.

4. *Heroin addict:* an individual who is physically and psychologically dependent on the narcotic drug, heroin.

5. *Ex-heroin addict:* an individual who is no longer physically and psychologically dependent on heroin.

   a. *Relapsed:* an addict who has begun to use heroin again on a regular basis at least once a day, who is readdicted, and who has again presented for treatment.

   b. *Unrelapsed:* an ex-addict who has remained abstinent.

6. *"Clean":* abstinent. *See also* Period of Abstinence.

Research Design

Introduction

This investigation will be a descriptive survey, based on a questionnaire and yielding interval data. The study will be retrospective rather than predictive. The plan consists of two major stages: the first is construction of the instrument, and the second, the selection of a sample, collection of the data, and data analysis.

Stage I: Creation of the Instrument

The original plan for collecting data was to use the existing SRE of Hawkins, Davies, and Holmes and Rahe. However, three interesting problems emerged in the preparation of this proposal, which have weighed heavily in the decision to construct a new tool.

Rationale for the Construction of a New Questionnaire

1. The SRRQ, published widely, contains several items which do not apply to unemployed heroin addicts, many of whom are stealing, borrowing, and using all of their personal resources to feed their habit. Items such as "Taking on a mortgage greater than $10,000" simply do not make sense to most of the study population in terms of their own lives (for the original SRRQ, see Appendix A). The SRE has not been published at all (Holmes and Masuda, 1974, p. 57). Dr. Holmes has invited inquiries regarding the cost and use of the SRE, and a letter has been sent to him (see Appendix B).

2. Since the construction of the original questionnaire, a growing number of investigators have used lists of stressful life events in order to study episodes of physical illness and psychological disorder. Some have used original lists, created for the population under study, some have used a preexisting list, and some a combination of the two.

3. Komaroff, Masuda, and Holmes found, in 1967, that members of two American subculture groups in Los Angeles—poor blacks and poor Mexican-Americans—rated the items on the SRRQ significantly differently from the White, middle class subjects of Holmes and Rahe. Additionally, they found some language which, on trial runs, was not understood by many respondents, and they changed the language of the items and the rating instructions (Komaroff, et al., 1968).

The SRE-SRQQ, Revised for the Study Population

The first step in designing the questionnaire was to ask as many people as possible—relapsed and unrelapsed addicts alike—the following question: What big changes in your life happened after you kicked (or after you kicked last time)? A probe was used if a person said, "None." This was the following question: For instance, did anything happen with your family, your friends, a job, or your place to live? Twenty people were interviewed in this manner. There were several items mentioned which were not on Holmes and Rahe's questionnaire, although many of them were the same. Also, respondents were asked to look over the list and to say which ones were valid and which were not, for people like themselves. The new questionnaire is presented below. It is designed to elicit from subjects their life change events during the current (or just past) period of abstinence. Items are either from the original SRRQ or are those which were generated by questioning members of the study population. Dr. Rahe or Dr. Holmes will be asked to critique the instrument. It will be called "The Significant Life Events Questionnaire."

Scaling

Three groups will be asked to rate the items on the questionnaire, so that the questionnaires can be scored for the data analysis. The groups will be the residents of Tu'um Est, a therapeutic community for drug abusers in Venice; Via Avante, a halfway house for drug abusers in Palms (residents live and work outside); and the members of the Friday night outpatient counseling group at the Venice Drug Coalition. The total number of people will be approximately 120. The instructions for the respondents come directly from Komaroff, et al., and are a modification of the original format used on a convenience sample of 394 respondents by Holmes and Rahe in 1967. The method for scaling was deprived from psychophysics, the division of psychology that deals with the human being's ability to make subjective magnitude estimations about certain of his experiences. The instructions will be given verbally.

Testing for Validity and Reliability of the Instrument

Validity: 1. A panel of eight judges will be assembled: four unrelapsed ex-addicts (two male, two female) who are working in the drug abuse field as counselors, and four relapsed ex-addicts (two male, two female), who have presented for treatment, to evaluate and critique the instrument.

2. A pretest on a pilot population of fifteen relapsed and unrelapsed individuals will be done, by interviewing in depth about their personal life change events, and then administering the questionnaire to them (Rahe, 1974).

Reliability: Following Rahe, test-retest will be the method of testing reliability. All individuals in the pilot study will be asked to participate. For Holmes and Rahe's original questionnaire, reliability estimates have ranged from .90 to .26. The dramatic differences are related to time interval between administrations (from two weeks to two years), educational level of the subjects, time interval over which recent life changes are summed, wording and format of the questions, and intercorrelations between various life change events (Rahe, 1974). For this pilot study, retest will be done in two weeks, simply because it's difficult to know where the relapsed addicts will be, even for that long.

Stage II: The Sample, Data Collection, Data Analysis

The Sample

A combination quota/purposive nonprobability sample will be used in this study. A sample will be drawn from each of two populations: ex-heroin addicts who have relapsed, and ex-heroin addicts who have not, all of whom have been abstinent for at least one year. The relapsed sample will be the first thirty individuals who present at the Venice Drug Coalition, a clearing house and intake service for a variety of treatment programs in the Venice-Santa Monica-West Los Angeles area, and as far away as detoxification units in hospitals in the San Fernando Valley. These clients come primarily from Los Angeles and Orange counties. The sex of the subjects is important for the study since some of the literature indicates that relapse patterns are different for males and females (Vaillant, 1966). However, several months of observation has indicated that there are sufficient numbers of both women and men that meet the criterion for the study to eliminate concern about disproportionate numbers.

The unrelapsed sample will be thirty individuals who have remained abstinent up until the time of the study. The selection will be made by word of mouth; individuals known to the investigator, others known to them, and so on in a widening circle. This method, totally purposive, is necessary in order to fulfill the needs of the study, since unrelapsed ex-addicts are really quite scarce, and since there appears to be a network of people who know one another as the circle widens. There is strong interest in the project among those who have heard about it, and assistance has been offered.

Protection of Human Rights

Each subject will receive, individually, an explanation about the purpose and the nature of the study and about the questionnaire. They will be reassured about their anonymity, and they will be told that it's possible that something can be learned about why people relapse after they've gone through the trouble and pain of kicking. A form will be given to each subject to sign. All respondents will be asked if they have any questions before signing, and if they have difficulty reading the form, it will be read to them. The investigator will not be the witness for the signatures.

Data Collection

Each potential subject in each sample will be approached individually and asked to participate in the study. In addition to the information given under Protection of Human Rights, each person will be told that the questionnaire consists of 43 items which have to do with things that have happened in his/her life since she/he kicked (this statement will be modified for the relapsed group by the addition of the words "last time.") all questions will be carefully answered. Each subject will be asked to fill out the part of the questionnaire that will give important information about him or herself, without putting a name on it. The following demographic data will be solicited: age, sex, age that heroin was first used, how many years addicted, ethnic group (a checklist for black, Chicano, white, and other be specific), employed or unemployed and occupation, still clean or using drugs again (a checklist will be given to meet the criteria under Definition of Terms), how many times kicked altogether.

Data Analysis

Several techniques will be employed in the analysis of data. First, a table will be set up which will show the frequencies of each of the variables in the questionnaire by each of the two sample groups. In order to simplify the table, i.e., to make it less cumbersome and easier to read, items will be placed in the columns by their number on the questionnaire rather than writing out the item in its entirety. For example, the item "Major change in eating habits (a lot more or a lot less food, or very different meal hours or kind of food or place where you eat)," the number 7 will be used in the column.

Two other tables will be constructed. One will assign all items on the SLEQ into four categories: family, work, personal, and financial. These categories were created by Rahe and his associates for a comparative study reported in 1971, in order to identify the nature of various life changes (Rahe, et al., 1971). For the present study, the purpose of the categorizations is to determine if some kinds of life change events occur more frequently than others in each of the two samples. Does either of the two groups have more family changes, or personal or work or financial changes?

The other table will assign all items to one of two categories: those indicative of life style of the individual, and those indicative of occurrences that involve the individual (after Holmes and Masuda, 1974). As with the preceding table, a chart will be made with each category heading at the top and the pertinent items listed beneath it.

Depending on the number and type of responses to Item 43, other categories will be set up and responses can be tabulated; or perhaps, at least for Table III and Table IV, the responses can fit into pre-existing categories.

In addition to frequency tables, each subject's questionnaire will be scored on the basis of the value (Life Change Unit) given to the item when the questionnaire was scaled. An arithmetic mean will be calculated for each group.

Keeping in mind that random sampling was not done for this study and that therefore no assumptions about representativeness can be made, and also keeping in mind that the design is not experimental and no hypotheses have been introduced, a t-test nevertheless seems appropriate with this interval data in order to determine if the means of the two groups differ significantly or if they differ only within the bounds of chance fluctuation. The t-test might be useful in the context of discovery. A significant difference will be reflected in the t-ratio by a statistic equal to or greater than 2.045 in a two-tailed test, with $n - 1 =$ 29 (df) at the .05 level of significance.

Limitations of the Study

1. The samples are small and are not necessarily representative of the universe of addicts and ex-addicts, and therefore no generalizations can be made. Not only are they small, but they are not probability samples.
2. The population of relapsed ex-addicts who have not sought further treatment is unavailable.
3. The data focus strictly on life change events and do not concern themselves with the ways in which these events are mediated by physiological or intrapsychic processes or by early conditioning.
4. The professional status, SES, and educational level of the investigator and her impersonal, rather than personal, knowledge of addiction may create mistrust and thereby alter results, in spite of her familiarity with the setting and culture and her efforts to help subjects be at ease. This problem may be mitigated somewhat by the fact that she has come to know and be comfortable with the population and they with her, and also that relationships of openness are already established.
5. No dividing lines between scores which indicate relapse and those that indicate no relapse have as yet been defined, and therefore they have no meaning except as those of relapsed and unrelapsed individuals relate to each other.

Interpretation of Results and Implications for Further Study

It is difficult to interpret results without data, but a few ideas are generated by the type of data to be collected and the data analysis plan:
1. Results can be interpreted on the basis of which (if either) of the two groups have higher frequencies in the categories of the tables.
2. Demographic data can also be analyzed; that is, the effect of age, sex, age of heroin debut, etc., on relapse can be explored, as well as the life change events.
3. An hypothesis about the effects of life change events, or certain categories of them, on relapse into addiction, may flow from this descriptive study.
4. The classifying of "desirable" and "undesirable" events by subjects, when and if the study is refined and redone, would add some information to the ongoing debate over what kinds of events are crucial in triggering illness, psychological problems, or in this case, relapse into addiction.

HOW TO SUCCEED IN GRADUATE SCHOOL
A RESEARCH PROPOSAL

Co-Principal Investigators:
Pamela J. Brink
Barbara A. Clemence
Marilynn J. Wood

How to Succeed in Graduate School

Eighty percent of all registered nurses in the United States have received their basic nursing education from an associate degree program or from a hospital school of nursing (1). These nurses, wishing to further their nursing education, find that there are relatively few schools of nursing available for them to continue their education and receive a Bachelor's degree in nursing. Yet the National League for Nursing has stated in its accreditation guide that the major criteria for entrance into a Master's degree program in nursing is graduation from an accredited Bachelor's program in nursing (2). As a result, many RNs have had to seek further education outside of nursing, and some have never returned to the profession. The dilemma lies in the fact that nursing needs academically trained individuals as teachers, as administrators, and as researchers—but is unable to utilize them due to its own mandate.

Many nursing educators have been disputing the mandate that only nurses from Bachelor's programs in nursing can be admitted to graduate programs in nursing (Lenburg and Yeaworth, 1975). The dispute arises from the fact that there is no proof available that there is a difference between nurses with nursing Bachelors and nurses with other Bachelor's degrees. And without that proof—some documented facts—these educators have insisted that some studies be done that will settle the argument once and for all.

Another basic disagreement lies in the philosophy of education. Many nurse educators believe that no matter what characteristics the student enters a program with, the end result should be the same, since it is the task of educational programs and educators to develop criteria for graduation and to offer curricula to achieve those criteria. Others believe that entrance characteristics are more critical to the program, and that anyone acceptable for entrance should be able to complete the program of studies. For these educators, anyone entering a program is guaranteed graduation unless the student drops out. Neither philosophical position has been challenged in nursing—both are in current operation across the country. But beliefs and philosophies are challengable and can be tested.

Other than philosphies of education, a second argument exists in relation to entrance versus exit competencies. This argument specifically relates to the realities of economics. Many educators believe that although, altruistically, the profession needs academically prepared nurses, the budgetary requirements of the school and/or the program cannot afford to maintain students beyond a certain length of time. These educators are of the opinion that relaxed admissions criteria result in more faculty time and longer tenure for students in the program and are therefore not feasible economically. Other nursing educators believe that the time and money are worth the development of nurses to assume positions of leadership within the profession. Neither position has been proven. There is no documentation that the RN with a Bachelor's degree in a field other than nursing takes more time to complete a graduate program than the RN with a nursing Bachelor's.

To date, the only study reported on graduate programs accepting nurses from various Bachelors' preparation is the study by Lenburg and Yeaworth (1975), yet this study was simply a survey of how many schools accepted RNs with other Bachelor's degrees and how these schools dealt with these students. Lenburg and Yeaworth raised the issues previously mentioned, that there is no proof of what constitutes nursing competencies, there are no methods of evaluating these competencies, and there is no discrimination between entrance and exit criteria. The study, in fact, raised the same issues that have been raised in the UCLA School of Nursing.

Because there is no documented proof of what constitutes a professional nurse versus what constitutes a technical nurse (3); because there is no documentation of methods of assessing exit competencies in graduate programs of nursing; and because there's no differentiation made between levels of competencies of Master's degree holders from nursing education programs, the faculty of the UCLA School of Nursing decided to test these ideas on a very beginning exploratory basis.

An exploratory study was designed to test the differences between graduate students admitted with a Bachelor's degree in a natural or social science and graduate students admitted with an accredited Bachelor's degree in nursing. The study began in the Spring of 1973 with the admission of one student having a Bachelor's degree in psychology and basic nursing education from an associate degree program. At the time the study began, no exit criteria were established other than successful completion of the program as defined by graduating from the program and receiving the Master's degree in nursing.

Yet no student admitted under this "experimental graduate admissions program" (4) has been unsuccessful as defined. All have completed the program of studies and received the degree. The result of this initial exploration was grossly inadequate to answer the question. Something was obviously wrong either with the question asked or in the discrimination between variables.

The concept of success, as used in the initial study, was defined as 1) meeting the requirements for the degree and 2) graduation. Since all experimental admissions students met the requirement for success, a more definitive definition was called for. However, the definition could be applied to all students admitted to the graduate program— not just the experimental group—and both the program and the students could be evaluated on the same scale for success. Indeed, just looking at the experimental group alone, without some baseline documentation from the regular admission students, was judged to be bad research and very poor program evaluation. In fact, some discrimination between the "barely-skim-by" graduate, the "average" graduate and the "honors" graduate could provide some beginning definition of "degrees of success" between and among graduate students.

For these reasons, a second study is being proposed to attempt to discriminate more definitively between the successful degree recipient and contrast the characteristics of the successful graduate to the unsuccessful graduate—the student who did not receive the degree.

Although the general definition of success remains the same— completion of the requirements for the degree and graduation—the definition of success also includes the degree to which the degree candidate met the requirements for graduation. Was the student a marginal student throughout the program? Was the student an average achiever? Was the student outstanding throughout the program? To what degree did the student achieve the goals and objectives of the Master's program as listed in the announcements of the school of nursing?

Since the UCLA School of Nursing has as its primary aim the preparation of the professional clinical nurse specialist, to what degree did the graduate achieve that primary aim? Is the graduate a "professional" as defined by the school? Can the student demonstrate the knowledge, skills, and competencies required by the school for the title "clinical specialist"? What are the differences between students who succeed and those who don't succeed? If these questions could be answered, then a beginning differentiation may be made between the technically competent graduate and the professional nurse clinician.

In addition to the primary aim of the school, the graduate student is expected to have knowledge and skills in research including the "analysis, articulation and documentation of the nursing process." To what extent was the graduate student able to demonstrate this capability? Did the student select the thesis option or take the comprehensive examination on research? In either case, was the research problem selected a problem involving the nursing process? How well did the graduate achieve the aim of the school—if at all?

For the purposes of this study, therefore, the concept of success has been expanded to include "the degree to which the graduate of the program met the requirements for the degree and the aims and objectives of the graduate program in nursing."

Purpose of the Study

The purpose of this study is to answer the question, what are the differences between students who succeed and those who don't succeed in the Master's program at the UCLA School of Nursing?

Definition of Terms

1. *Succeed:* The degree to which the graduate of the UCLA School of Nursing met the requirements for the degree and the goals of the graduate program, as evidenced from student records.
2. *Degree of success:* Differentiates between 1) high achiever, 2) average achiever, 3) marginal achiever, and 4) non-achiever, (or the student who does not succeed), as demonstrated by the student records.
3. *High achiever:* The graduate who completed all requirements for the degree within six quarters or less; completed a thesis on a clinical nursing problem or achieved a score of 5 on the two clinical nursing questions in the comprehensive examinations in addition to a score of 5 on the research question in comprehensive examinations and took the examination only once; achieved a grade of A on all clinical course work (i.e., 420 and 470); maintained a 3.0 grade point average for every quarter of the graduate program.
4. *Average achiever:* The graduate who completed all requirements for the degree within six quarters or less; who wrote a thesis or achieved at least a score of three on the clinical and research questions and passed the comprehensive examination the first time taken; achieved at least a grade of B in all clinical course work; and maintained a 3.0 grade point average for every quarter of the graduate program.
5. *Marginal achiever:* The graduate who completed all requirements for the degree; who wrote a thesis or eventually passed

comprehensive examinations by achieving at least a score of 3 on both the clinical and research questions; maintained an overall grade point average of 3.0 although may have been on academic probation one or more times (does not include admission on probation).

6. *Non-achiever:* Did not complete requirements for the degree as specified above.

7. *Non-success:* Does not meet any of the above criteria for success.

8. *Differences:* The degree recipient will have evidence in student records of demographic data, admissions materials, progress through the curriculum, comprehensive examination scores or thesis data, in order to meet the criteria of success/non-success.

9. *Demographic data:* Whatever data available in the student record on such matters as: age, sex, ethnic group or nationality, number of years in nursing practice, field of practice and years in each field, number of years since obtaining Bachelor's degree, number of years since taking any academic courses, number of years since basic nursing education.

10. *Admission materials:* The degree recipient will have in student files evidence of: quarter and year admitted; GPA on admission for total program and for major field (post-graduate if available); name of major field for the Bachelor's degree; type of basic nursing education (diploma, ADN, BSN); admission on probation, deficiencies (number and type); differences between graduate admissions documentation and school of nursing admissions records on any and all of the above.

11. *Progress through the curriculum:* The degree recipient will have evidence of: number of times on probation; number of drop/add petitions and for what courses; grades on individual course work; GPA each quarter and overall cumulative GPA; number of times repeated clinical courses and which courses; changes in clinical areas including quarter of change and number of times changed; number of courses in declared functional area; number of other functional courses taken and of which type; number of credits accrued on graduation; number of electives outside of nursing and in which departments; number of quarters to complete program; number of courses transferred for degree; number of independent study courses and which; number of incompletes on transcripts and which courses; number of quarters on leave of absence and for what reasons; quarter dropped program;

financial aid—type and duration; thesis option—completed; comprehensive examination option—completed; number of times taking comprehensive examinations; scores on individual questions in comprehensive examinations.

12. *Goals of the graduate program:* As specified in the School of Nursing announcement, there is a central goal of clinical specialist, research as a secondary goal, and functional preparation as an option.

13. *Primary goal:* States the professional nurse specialist has an extensive body of nursing knowledge and a high level of competence in a specialized area of nursing and a field of clinical practice. Student demonstrates level of achievement of this goal through grades in clinical courses (A-B-C-F-dropped) and scores on the clinical question on comprehensives (0-1-2-3-4-5).

14. *Secondary goal:* States that the clinical nurse specialist is capable of utilizing the research process including analysis articulation and documentation of the nursing process. Student demonstrates the level of achievement of this goal through grades in research courses (A-B-C-F-dropped), scores on the research question on comprehensive examinations (0-1-2-3-4-5) and if a thesis was written, if that thesis were research on the clinical process.

15. *Optional goal:* States that the professional nurse specialist has knowledge and skill in functional areas of teaching, consultation and supervision as an elective. Student demonstrates the level of achievement of this goal through grades in functional courses, if taken (A-B-C-F-dropped), scores on the functional question in comprehensive examinations if taken (0-1-2-3-4-5), and content of the thesis if used as that option.

16. *Thesis option:* If the student did not write a thesis, a score of 9 (does not apply) will be given. If a student does write a thesis, the student will be given a score of 5, if the thesis were on the nursing process, a score of 4 for a functional topic (if the student also took elective courses in that functional area), and a score of 3 if the thesis did not meet either of these criteria.

Study Design

The study design is a historical evaluative research survey of all possible variables that may or may not affect the terminal criteria of program completion and passing comprehensive examinations or approval of a thesis, and achievement of the goals of the graduate program. The methods of data collection require a total population and available data. This study will be limited to an analysis of the differences between available data on admission criteria and the successful/nonsuccessful outcomes of program completion, comprehensive examinations, thesis, and achievement of the goals.

The sample population will include all students entering the Master's program in the UCLA School of Nursing from Spring, 1973, through Spring, 1975.

The School of Nursing, housed on a general state university campus, accepts students into the nursing program each quarter: Fall, Winter and Spring. Candidates for the Master's of Nursing degree are required to meet general university requirements for admission and graduation, over and above the professional curricula required by the School of Nursing. One exception to the admission requirements in the School of Nursing was the acceptance of nurses with a Bachelor's degree in another field than Nursing. The degree in the other field must be closely related to nursing, e.g., the behavioral and basic sciences.

Methods of Data Collection

Available data from student folders housed in the School of Nursing will be transcribed onto a tally sheet by a research assistant. The student folders include information on: courses taken and grades received, academic probation, demographic data, computed grade point averages, and letters of reference. Data will be collected in February, 1977. Computer cards will be keypunched by the University Computer Facility keypunch operators.

Data Analysis

Raw data will be subjected to measures of central tendency, chi-square and cross-tabulation. Further analyses of any significant results from any of the above will be made.

Additional Bibliography

Abdellah, F. G., and Levine, E. *Better Patient Care through Nursing Research.* New York: Macmillan Co., 1965.

American Nurses Association. *Report of Nursing Research Conferences.* Division of Nursing, N.I.H., U.S.P.H.S., 1965–1973.

Babbie, E. P. *Survey Research Methods.* Belmont, Calif.: Wadsworth Publishing Co., 1973.

Batey, Marjorie V., ed. *Communicating Nursing Research.* Vol. 1–10. Western Interstate Commission for Higher Education, Boulder, Colorado, 1968–1977.

Campbell, Donald T., and Stanley, Julian C. *Experimental and Quasi Experimental Designs for Research.* Chicago: Rand McNally, 1963.

Downs, Florence S., and Newman, Margaret A. *A Sourcebook of Nursing Research.* Philadelphia: F. A. Davis Co., 1973.

Festinger, L., and Katz, D. *Research Methods in the Behavioral Sciences.* New York: The Dryden Press, 1953.

Fox, D. J. *Fundamentals of Research in Nursing.* New York: Appleton-Century-Crofts, 1970.

Glaser, Barney G., and Strauss, Anselm L. *The Discovery of Grounded Theory: Strategies for Qualitative Research.* Chicago: Aldine Press, 1967.

Kerlinger, F. N. *Foundations of Behavioral Research.* 2d ed. New York: Holt, Rinehart and Winston, Inc., 1973.

Levitt, E. E. *Clinical Research Design and Analysis.* Springfield, Ill.: Charles C. Thomas, Publisher, 1961.

Lindzey, G., and Aronson, E. *The Handbook of Social Psychology.* 5 vols. Menlo Park, Calif.: Addison-Wesley Publishing Co., 1968.

Miller, Delbert C. *Handbook of Research Design and Social Measurement.* 2d ed. New York: David McKay Co., 1970.

Notter, Lucille. *Essentials of Nursing Research.* New York: Springer Publishing Co., 1974.

Pelto, Pertti J. *Anthropological Research: The Structure of Inquiry.* New York: Harper & Row, 1970.

Phillips, B. S. *Social Research Strategy and Tactics.* New York: Macmillan Co., 1968.

Phillips, J. L. *Statistical Thinking.* San Francisco: Freeman & Co., 1973.

Phillips, J. S., and Thompson, R. F. *Statistics for Nurses.* New York: Macmillan Co., 1967.

Reeder, Leo G., Ramacher, Linda, and Gorelnik, Sally. *Handbook of Scales and Indices of Health Behavior.* Santa Monica, Calif.: Goodyear Publishing Co., 1976.

Schatzman, L., and Strauss, A. L. *Field Research.* Englewood Cliffs, N.J.: Prentice-Hall, 1973.

Selltiz, Claire, Lawrence S. Wrightsman, and Stuart W. Cook. *Research Methods in Social Relations.* 3d ed. New York: Holt, Rinehart and Winston, 1976.

Siegel, S. *Nonparametric Statistics for the Behavioral Sciences.* New York: McGraw-Hill Book Co., 1956.

Treece, E. W. and Treece, J. W. *Elements of Research in Nursing.* St. Louis: C. V. Mosby Co., 1973.

Wandelt, M. *Guide for the Beginning Researcher.* New York: Appleton-Century-Crofts, 1970.

Wax, Rosalie H. *Doing Fieldwork: Warnings and Advice.* Chicago: The University of Chicago Press, 1971.

Weiss, Carol H. *Evaluation Research: Methods of Assessing Program Effectiveness.* Englewood Cliffs, N.J.: Prentice-Hall, Inc., 1972.

Some Further Suggestions

Books, like research proposals, are conceptualized and written in a certain order. Often, second thoughts occur during the writing of the book that don't really fit anywhere in the manuscript. Yet, those second thoughts have some value. We had a number of "second thoughts" while writing this book, and since we wanted to write a practical guide to planning a research project, we thought we should add them to the book.

The next pages are thoughts that occurred to us while lecturing in class, reading over the manuscript, or correcting papers. Some of these additions are for emphasis, others for practicality. We couldn't find them anywhere except in conversations, but feel that you might find them useful.

Literature Review. When you are looking up your topic initially, don't hesitate to look in theory, history, or even fictional literature for material on your idea. Sometimes there is not much available in the research literature, but a great deal in other sources. Use any source available on your topic and check it for accuracy.

Be sure to check sources both in and out of nursing. Sometimes the literature in the area is found only in history books or books on sociology. Check the various professional indexes for sources, look up synonyms and antonyms and check those out, talk to people and ask them to help you think of sources for your search. Don't hesitate to use any source you can find that substantiates your topic. Since nursing is an eclectic field and has built its knowledge on an amalgam of ideas outside of its major areas of interest, the breadth of reading possible for any topic is enormous.

Remember that good research is ethical research. If you say that there is no prior research in an area, then you will be believed. Your word of honor is accepted until proven to be otherwise. Your statements are accepted at face value. If you say you have done your literature review, you will be believed.

A major problem that crops up over and over again is losing your references. Be sure to keep a record of everything you have read about your topic and put it somewhere that you can find it until after you have finished the research project in its entirety. Don't throw away your bibliography cards—you never know when you will need them. You can be absolutely sure that if you lose, misplace, or throw away one bibliography card, that is the one you will desperately need when you write your proposal.

Applicability of Findings.   Research is usable only for the person who reads it. This is true simply because the person who reads the research knows its strengths and weaknesses on the basis of the critical review. The reader, therefore, is also the person who will apply the findings.

Applicability refers to a whole gamut of activities in addition to further research in the area. When we know the side effects of a particular level of medication dosage, then we can reduce the amount if we wish to decrease the side effects. If we know that increased age effects length of convalescence, we can plan for longer periods of convalescence. If we know that certain types of patients adversely affect the nursing staff, we can alter the nurses attitudes, alter the patient type, or simply make everyone aware of the situation.

When you are reading research reports for the applicability of the findings, look at your own professional practice—can use be made of this information in clinical practice, in educational settings, in administrative functions, in different age groups? *Applicability* means *use*.

And finally, remember that applicability refers to the use of research to further our knowledge base—and that pure and applied research are simply different types of research that are usable in nursing. Simply because research is usable does not make it applied; pure research is also usable.

Replication Research.   Replicate some one else's research if that's what you really want to do. Replication studies are absolutely necessary in knowledge-building, so don't drop a replication idea if its a good one —any more than you would drop any other research idea you had. But remember: you must have just as good a reason for a replication study —a good rationale—as for any other kind.

A second point to remember for replication is that only the sample changes. Nothing else can change in this type of design.

Resources.   When we get busy or pressured, we tend to forget the resources available to us in our research. Use your reference librarian as much as you need to—that's what a librarian is for. Don't hesitate simply because you aren't sure you know what to look for—ask for help.

A second area of resources is *money*. Don't hesitate to seek out funding sources and ask for monetary assistance if you need it. No one is going to offer you money if you don't express a need or desire for it. Your library or administration office has books that can assist you in this search. Use them.

Level of Research Design. Remember that the level of research design is indicative of the amount of information known about the topic and variables. The level *does not* refer to the level of research expertise of the researcher. Therefore, *do not* select a level one question simply because you are a novice, when your topic really calls for a level 2 or 3 question.

Write and rewrite your research question over and over again until you have the question exactly the way you want it. Don't be satisfied with a sloppy question. If the question is not clear to anyone else—rewrite it. If you find yourself saying, "Well, I know what I mean," then you are not being specific and clear.

In double-checking your question for level and clarity look for the following:

1. If your question has *cause* in it, look for the *effects* and vice versa.
2. If your question has either *cause* or *effects,* you are in level III.
3. Don't write a *why* question unless you know the effect of a variable.
4. Don't write an *if-then* question unless you know the *cause* variable.
5. Don't write either a level I or level II question if you are questioning causes and effects.

Research and Writing Go Together. Don't expect anyone to approve your research proposal until you have written it out. The most you can get for your idea is verbal encouragement until the proposal is written.

On the other hand, don't write the proposal as a finished project until you have checked it thoroughly. Make sure that every part of the proposal is consistent with every other part of the proposal. Again, if you have a *why* question as your base, you must have an hypothesis. If you have a *why* question and a declarative statement and content analysis, you are probably not finished with your plan.

Remember to be specific in everything you say. Every word needs to be described in such a way that it can be measured or observed. If you use a word such as *loss,* be specific about what *you* mean by *loss.* Don't hunt up someone else's definition. Think how you want to measure loss, and what kind of loss you are measuring. Many people confuse loss and grief because they do not read their own definitions of these terms.

Don't confuse vagueness with sophistication.
Don't use three-syllable words when a two-syllable word is clearer.

Be Assertive!   Develop your own idea for research. Don't let others talk you out of your idea, or intimidate you, or tell you that you should research their idea instead. At the same time, make sure you know what you are talking about; otherwise, anyone can talk you out of anything.

Practice Deferred Gratification.   Although its a severe temptation, *don't* start collecting data before you have written out your research plan and had it approved for the protection of human rights.

In the same vein, don't analyze available data before you have finished your proposal. Until you know what answers you are looking for, you are simply wasting your time. And until you have written it all out in the form of a proposal, you have no idea just how fuzzy your thinking really is.

So write your proposal before going on to the other phases of research.

Index